GUIDELINES FOR
DESIGN AND
CONSTRUCTION OF

1996-97

HOSPITAL
AND
HEALTH CARE
FACILITIES

■ The American Institute of Architects Academy
of Architecture for Health with assistance from
the U.S. Department of Health and Human Services

The American Institute of Architects Press
WASHINGTON, D.C.

The American Institute of Architects Press
1735 New York Avenue, N.W.
Washington, D.C. 20006

ISBN 1-55835-151-5

CONTENTS

Tables

PREFACE

This is the latest in a 45-year series of guidelines to aid in the design and construction of hospital and medical facilities.

The original *General Standards* appeared in the *Federal Register* on February 14, 1947, as part of the implementing regulations for the Hill-Burton program. The standards were revised from time to time as needed. In 1973, the document was retitled Minimum Requirements of Construction and Equipment for Medical Facilities to emphasize that the requirements were generally minimum, rather than recommendations of ideal standards.

Sections 603(b) and 1620(2) of the Public Health Service Act require the Secretary of the Department of Health and Human Services (HHS) to prescribe by regulation general standards of construction, renovation, and equipment for projects assisted under Title VI and Title XVI, respectively, of the act. Since Title VI and Title XVI grant and loan authorities have expired, there is no need to retain the standards in regulation.

In 1984, HHS removed from regulation the requirements relating to minimum standards of construction, renovation, and equipment of hospitals and other medical facilities, as cited in the *Minimum Requirements,* DHEW Publication No. (HRA) 81-14500. To reflect the nonregulatory status, the title was changed to *Guidelines for Construction and Equipment of Hospital and Medical Facilities.* For this 1996–97 edition, the title has been amended to read *Guidelines for Design and Construction of Hospital and Health Care Facilities* to reflect the scope, content, and usage of this document.

These *Guidelines* are evolving in order to provide guidance to providers, designers, and regulators in a continually changing environment. It is recognized that many health care services may be provided in facilities not subject to licensure or regulation, and it is intended that these *Guidelines* be suitable for use by all health care providers. It is further intended that, when used as regulations, some latitude be granted in complying with these *Guidelines,* so long as the health and safety of the occupants of the facility are not compromised.

The *Guidelines* will be used by HHS to assess Department of Housing and Urban Development Section 242 applications for hospital mortgage insurance and the Indian Health Service construction projects. The *Guidelines* may also be used by other entities, such as state licensure agencies. For this reason, regulatory language was retained. The 1996–97 edition of the *Guidelines* follows these principles. Explanatory and guide material is included in appendix A, which is not mandatory.

The Health Care Finance Administration (HCFA) and the Health Resources Services Administration (HRSA), which are both in the Department of Health and Human Services, are supporting the efforts of the 1996–97 *Guidelines* both financially and with support staff. HCFA has the responsibility for the reimbursement and operation of the Medicare and Medicaid programs. Hospital construction and costs are directly related to the charge of HCFA's mission. Although HCFA is not adopting the *Guidelines* as regulations, the agency does concur with the design and construction recommendations.

This edition of the *Guidelines* reflects the work of advisory groups from private, state, and federal sectors, representing expertise in design, operation, and construction of health facilities. Advisory group members reviewed the 1992–93 edition of the *Guidelines* line by line, revising details as necessary to accommodate current health care procedures and to provide a desirable environment for patient care at a reasonable facility cost.

The *Guidelines* standards are performance oriented for desired results. Prescriptive measurements, where given, have been carefully considered relative to generally recognized standards and do not require detail specification. For example, experience has shown that it would be extremely difficult to design a patient bedroom smaller than the size suggested and have space for functions and procedures that are normally expected.

Authorities adopting the *Guidelines* standards should encourage design innovations and grant exceptions where the intent of the standards is met. These standards assume that appropriate architectural and engineering practice and compliance with applicable codes will be observed as part of normal professional service and require no separate detailed instructions.

In some facility areas or sections, it may be desirable to exceed the *Guidelines* standards for optimum function. For example, door widths for inpatient hospital rooms are noted as 3 feet 8 inches (1.11 meters), which satisfies most applicable codes, to permit passage of patient beds. However, wider widths of 3 feet 10 inches (1.16 meters) or even 4 feet (1.22 meters) may be desirable to reduce damage to doors and frames where frequent movement of beds and large equipment may occur. The decision to exceed the standards should be made by the individuals involved.

In many ways, the *Guidelines* may be considered a consensus document. There have been at least two national reviews by all interest groups, and by state and federal entities. While the *Guidelines* started as a federal document, the American Institute of Architects has made it a national document to improve the health of the nation.

This publication supersedes DHHS Publication Nol (HRS-M-HF) 84-1, DHEW Publication No. (HRA) 79-14500, DHEW Publication No. (HRA) 76-4000, the 1992–93 edition of the *Guidelines*.

Inquiries or questions on the *Guidelines* may be addressed to the following groups:

American Institute of Architects
Academy of Architecture for Health
1735 New York Avenue, N.W.
Washington, D.C. 20006

Health Resources and Services Administration
Division of Facilities Loans
5600 Fishers Lane, Room 11A-14
Rockville, Maryland 20857

Office of Engineering Services
Region II
Room 3309
26 Federal Plaza
New York, New York 10278

MAJOR ADDITIONS AND REVISIONS

To reflect the scope, content, and usage of this document, the previous title has been amended to *Guidelines for Design and Construction of Hospital and Health Care Facilities* for this 1996–97 edition.

The format and technical content, in general, follow the previous document, *Guidelines for Construction and Equipment of Hospital and Medical Facilities, 1992–93 Edition*. The exception to this is that elevators will always be section 30.B (i.e., 7.30.B, 8.30.B, 9.30.B, etc.); waste processing will be 30.C, HVAC 31.A through D, plumbing 31.E, electrical 32.A through F, nurses call 32.G, emergency electrical service 32.H, fire alarm system 32.J, and telecommunications 32.J. Appendix B has been eliminated. All significant changes are identified by a vertical line in the margin. An asterisk (*) preceding a number or letter designating a paragraph indicates explanatory material about that paragraph can be found in appendix A.

Many editorial changes were made to correct errors or inconsistencies or to clarify the intent. Listed below are major additions and revisions made to this edition of the *Guidelines.*

1. Infection control

Significant changes have been incorporated into these *Guidelines* with regard to infection control, types of isolation requirements, and ventilation. To every extent possible, these changes conform to the most current Centers for Disease Control and Prevention "Guidelines for Preventing the Transmission of Mycobacterium Tuberculosis in Health Care Facilities" and "Guidelines for Prevention of Nosocomial Pneumonia, 1994." Three patient segregation categories have been identified:

- Airborne infection isolation room

- Protective environment room

- Immunosuppressed host in airborne infection isolation

A new process called "infection control risk assessment" is introduced to describe how an organization determines the risk for transmission of various infectious pathogens. This process is an essential component of any facility's functional or master programming, since there may be significant differences in population. This organizational committee should be a multidisciplinary panel with expertise in areas of infectious disease, facility design and construction, ventilation and epidemiology, etc. The purpose of this committee is to coordinate the individual infection control needs of the organization with the appropriate numbers and types of isolation rooms and procedure rooms. It is the intent of this process to allow flexibility in meeting individual organizational needs for creating a safer environment for patients, staff, and visitors.

Anteroom space in either airborne infection isolation or protective environment rooms is no longer required. Anterooms are recommended only for those organizations with patients who are both immunosuppressed and potential transmitters of airborne infection. Anterooms are also required in those facilities in which the infection control risk assessment dictates the need for special operating suites and delivery rooms.

Rooms with dual-purpose or switch-reversible airflow mechanisms that allow rooms to be switched between positive and negative pressure configurations are no longer acceptable.

2. Section 5.1, Construction Phasing, has been completely changed to reflect infectious hazards that may be encountered during health care facility planning, design, construction phasing, and commissioning, in addition to occupant safety and comfort.

3. Section 7.3.A.3. The minimum area permitted in renovation of existing critical care units has been increased from 120 square feet (11.15 square meters) to 130 square feet (12.09 square meters) for single-patient rooms (or cubicles) and from 100 square feet (9.29 square meters) to 110 square feet (10.23 square meters) per bed in multiple-bed space.

4. Sections 7.3.D.8 and 7.5.E, Examination and Treatment Rooms. Omitting these elements in pediatric critical care units and in pediatric and adolescent units is no longer permitted even if all patients are in private rooms.

5. Section 7.3.E.8. A new requirement has been added that each patient space in a newborn intensive care unit shall have a minimum of 100 square feet (9.29 square meters).

6. Section 7.6.C has been changed to require at least one airborne infection isolation room in the psychiatric unit.

7. Section 7.8.A2.a(3). Permission to continue in use existing three- or four-bed rooms in renovation projects has been deleted. All rooms must have two beds or fewer.

8. Section 7.9.D3. Triage areas in the emergency department must be designed and ventilated to reduce exposure of staff, patients, and families to airborne infectious diseases.

9. Sections 7.9.D3 and 7.10.G1. Waiting areas in the emergency department and in the imaging suite have been singled out as areas that may require special measures to reduce the risk of airborne infection transmission.

10. Sections 7.10.H1 through 7.10.H11, Cardiac Catheterization Lab, have been moved from the appendix to the body of the *Guidelines* and modified from recommendations to requirements.

11. Section 7.14, Renal Dialysis Unit, an entire new section, has been added.

12. Sections 7.30.B2 and 10.30.B1. The minimum size for hospital and rehabilitation elevator cars has been increased from 5 feet (1.52 meters) wide and 7 feet 6 inches (2.29 meters) deep to 5 feet 8 inches (1.73 meters) wide and 9 feet (2.74 meters) deep. A renovation exception has been added.

13. Section 7.31.D24. A new requirement has been added for rooms used for sputum induction, aerolized pentamidine treatments, and other high-risk areas.

14. Section 7.31.D25. A new paragraph has been added permitting fan coil and individual heating and cooling units in certain areas of the hospital provided that all outdoor air requirements shall be supplied by a central ventilation system that meets the filtration requirements in Table 3.

15. Sections 7.32.G, 8.32.G, 10.32.G, and 11.32.G, Nurses Calling Systems, have been changed to permit the use of new technologies such as radio frequency systems.

16. Table 2 has been changed to:

Add bronchoscopy and endoscopy requirements.

Change protective isolation to protective environment and increase total air changes from 6 to 12.

Change relative humidity in operating rooms and delivery rooms from 50–60 percent to 30–60 percent and temperature range from 70°–75°F (21°–24°C) to 68°–73°F (20°–23°C).

Change airborne infectious isolation room total air changes from 6 to 12.

Increase patient room outdoor air changes from 1 to 2.

Increase labor/delivery/recovery and LDRP outdoor air changes from 0 to 2.

Add a temperature requirement of 75°F (24°C) to general laboratory, biochemistry, histology, microbiology, nuclear medicine, pathology, and serology.

17. Table 3. The efficiency requirement for filter bed No. 1 has been increased from 25 percent to 30 percent.

18. Chapter 8 has been revised to reflect the changing mission and roles of nursing facilities. Sections on subacute care and Alzheimer's have been added.

19. Section 8.2.C1. Nurses station has been changed to staff work area and the text revised to permit alternative arrangements for centralized or decentralized caregiving.

20. Table 6 has been changed to add requirements for:

• Protective environment and airborne infectious isolation.

• Dining rooms and activity rooms.

21. Table 8. Maximum and minimum temperature requirements have been changed as follows:

Resident care areas: from maximum 110°F (43°C) to maximum 95°–110°F (35°–43°C).

Dietary: from minimum 120°F (49°C) to minimum 140°F (60°C).

Laundry: from minimum 160°F (71°C) to minimum 140°F (60°C).

22. Table 9, Illuminations Values for Nursing, has been deleted.

23. Sections 8.7, Subacute Care Facilities, and 13, Hospice Care, both have suggested text in the appendix in order to solicit public proposals to the Guidelines committee to develop minimum guidelines for the next edition.

24. Throughout all sections, handwashing facilities are now required in all toilet rooms. Permission to omit them under certain circumstances has been deleted.

25. A form for public proposals for future changes to the *Guidelines* is included.

ACKNOWLEDGMENTS

The Academy of Architecture for Health (AAH) of the American Institute of Architects (AIA) was privileged to convene and work with an interdisciplinary committee to revise the *Guidelines for Construction and Equipment of Hospital and Medical Facilities*. This is the third revision cycle for which the AIA/AAH has been honored to serve in this capacity. They played a major role in the preparation of this edition, entitled *Guidelines for Design and Construction of Hospital and Health Care Facilities*.

These revised Guidelines are the result of many hours of concentrated work by dedicated professionals concerned with the health care industry from private practice, professional organizations, and state and federal agencies. More than 2,000 proposals for change and comments on proposed changes were received and processed at three meetings held in Baltimore, San Diego, and Denver. Approximately 65 members attended each meeting and gave serious and full consideration to all written comments and proposals. The AIA wishes to express its sincere gratitude to all who sent comments and to those organizations whose representatives served on the Guidelines Revision Committee.

Steering Group

Joseph G. Sprague, FAIA
Chairman
HKS Architects, Inc.

Douglas S. Erickson, FASHE
Vice Chairman
American Hospital Association

J. Armand Burgun, FAIA
Chairman Emeritus
Rodgers Burgun Shahine
& Deschler

Michelle Donovan, R.N.
Ambulatory Care Advisory
Group, Inc.

Daniel L. Hightower, R.A.
U.S. Department of Health and
Human Services, NIH

Neil Kellman, M.D.
California Office of Statewide
Health Planning and Development

Todd S. Phillips, Ph.D., AIA
American Institute of Architects

Emilio M. Pucillo, R.A.
U.S. Department of Health and
Human Services, HRSA, OES

David A. Rhodes, FAIA
JMGR, Inc.

Ralph Swain, Ph.D.
Shands Hospital

Mayer Zimmerman
U.S. Department of Health and
Human Services, HCFA

Guidelines Revision Committee

James V. Allred, AIA
U.S. Army Corps of Engineers

Michael R. Arnold, AIA
Granary Associates

Donald E. Baptiste
Sturdy Memorial Hospital Inc.

Judene Bartley, M.S., M.P.H.
Harper Hospital

Chris Bettlach, P.E.
Sisters of Mercy Health System—
St. Louis

James R. Biasco, P.E.
U.S. Department of Health and
Human Services, IHS

Leon B. Boland, P.E.
Wisconsin State Division of Health

Brenda Bouvier
Association for Professionals in
Infection Control and Epidemiology

Mary Jo Breslin
University of Maryland Medical
Systems

George Byrns, R.S., MPH
U.S. Department of Health and
Human Services, IHS

Joseph W. Carobene, CMHA
Middle Tennessee MH Institute

Jack Chamblee
Healthsouth Corporation

Martin H. Cohen, FAIA
Forum for Health Care Planning

Walter Collins, P.E.
Parsons Brinckerhoff, Facilities
Services

Ed Denton, AIA
Kaiser Permanente

Scott J. Doellinger
Design Group, Inc.

John M. Dombrowski, P.E.
H. F. Lenz Company

Roger W. Gehrke
Idaho Department of Health
and Welfare

Marjorie Geist, R.N., M.S.N.,
M.H.A.
American College of Emergency
Physicians

Carole Gilmore, Lt. Col.
U.S. Army Health Facility
Planning Agency

Warren N. Goodwin, AIA
Quorom Health Resources, Inc.

Rita A. Gore, R.N.
New Jersey Department of Health

James R. Gregory
Agency for Healthcare Administration, Florida

Ken Gurtowski
Calumet Coach Company

Jill Hall
Institute for Family-Centered Care

Maureen Harvey, R.N.
Society of Critical Care Medicine

Robert Hughes
NIOSH

Thomas W. Jaeger, P.E.
Gage Babcock and Associates, Inc.

Dwight H. Jones, P.E.
Georgia Department of Human
Resources

Thomas M. Jung
New York State Department
of Health

Ode R. Keil, PE
SMS

Stuart L. Keill, M.D.
American Psychiatric Association

Carol Kershner
Episcopal Ministries to the Aging

Steve M. Lakner
Central DuPage Health System

Roger J. Langlois
Connecticut Department
of Public Health

Harold Laufman, M.D., Ph.D.
HLA Systems

James Lefter
University of Illinois

Terence G. Lewis Sr.
Association of Massachusetts
Homes for the Aging

Stephen G. Lynn, M.D., FACEP
American College of Emergency
Physicians

Charles E. Maher
Ochsner Medical Institutions

James Merrill
U.S. Department of Health
and Human Services, HCFA

Robert A. Michaels, Ph.D., CEP
RAM TRAC Health Risk Consultants of Schenectady, NY

Juanita Mildenberg, AIA
U.S. Department of Health and
Human Services, NIH

R. Gregg Moon, NCARB
Baylor College of Medicine,
Houston

Robert Mullan, M.D.
Centers for Disease Control-NIOSH

Dennis Murray
K.M.S. and Associates, Ltd.

Francis C. Nance, M.D.
American College of Surgeons

Hugh Nash, P.E.
Smith Seckman Reid Inc.

Paul Ninomura, P.E.
U.S. Department of Health and
Human Services, OES

Timothy M. Peglow, P.E., CCE,
SASHE
LaPorte Hospital, Inc.

Douglas Pendergras
Convalescent Enterprises, Inc.

Zenon A. Pihut, P.E.
Texas Department of Health

Gina Pugliese, R.N., M.S.
Sullivan Kelly & Associates, Inc.

Cheryl Riskin
HMR Associates

Kurt Rockstroh, AIA
SBA/Steffian Bradley Associates, Inc.

Chris Rousseau, P.E.
Newcomb & Boyd Consulting
Engineers

Arthur St. Andre, M.D.
Washington Hospital Center

Janet Schultz, R.N.
AMSCO International

William Sciarillo, Sc.D.
Association for the Care of
Children's Health

Lloyd H. Siegel, FAIA
U.S. Department of Veterans Affairs

David Sine, CSP
National Association of Psychiatric
Healthcare Systems

Grady Smith, Architect, AIA
Judith Smith

Smith Hager Bajo, Inc.
Maureen Smith
Centers for Disease Control
& Prevention

Joseph Strauss, AIA, CHC
Lammers + Gershon Assocs., Inc.
American Association of Healthcare
Consultants

Andrew J. Streifel, M.P.H.
University of Minnesota

Drexel Toland
Drexel Toland & Associates, Inc.

Marjorie Underwood, R.N.
Association for Professionals in
Infection Control and Epidemiology

Marjorie E. Vincent, R.N., MBA
Premier Ambulatory Systems

Kathryn D. Wagner, Ph.D.
Kathryn D. Wagner, Ph.D.

John A. Westcott
Northwestern Memorial Hospital

James H. Wilson
U.S. Department of Health and
Human Services, NIH

Special thanks are due to the Health Care Finance
Administration and the Health Resources and Services
Administration of the U.S. Department of Health and
Human Services, which provided major funding for
the project.

Joseph G. Sprague, FAIA
Chairman
Guidelines Revision Committee

1. INTRODUCTION

1.1 General

1.1.A.

This document contains information intended as minimum standards for constructing and equipping new health care facility projects. For brevity and convenience these standards are presented in "code language." Use of words such as *shall* is mandatory only where applied by an adopting authority having jurisdiction. Insofar as practical, these standards relate to desired performance or results or both. Details of construction and engineering are assumed to be part of good design practice and local building regulations. Design and construction shall conform to the requirements of these Guidelines. Requirements set forth in these Guidelines shall be considered as minimum. For aspects of design and construction not included in these Guidelines, local governing building codes shall apply. Where there is no local governing building code, the prevailing model code used within the geographic area is hereby specified for all requirements not otherwise specified in these Guidelines. (See Section 1.4 for wind and seismic local requirements.)

Where ASCE 7-93 is referenced, similar provisions in the model building code are considered substantially equivalent.

An asterisk (*) preceding a paragraph number indicates that explanatory or educational material can be found in Appendix A.

1.1.B.

This document covers health facilities common to communities in this country. Facilities with unique services will require special consideration. However, sections herein may be applicable for parts of any facility and may be used where appropriate.

1.1.C.

These Guidelines are not intended to restrict innovations and improvements in design or construction techniques. Accordingly, authorities adopting these standards as codes may approve plans and specifications which contain deviations if it is determined that the respective intent or objective has been met. Final implementation may be subject to requirements of the authority having jurisdiction.

1.1.D.

Some projects may be subject to the regulations of several different programs, including those of state, local, and federal authorities. While every effort has been made for coordination, individual project requirements should be verified, as appropriate. Should requirements be conflicting or contradictory, the authority having primary responsibility for resolution should be consulted.

1.1.E.

The Health Care Financing Administration, which is responsible for Medicare and Medicaid reimbursement, has adopted the National Fire Protection Association 101 Life Safety Code (NFPA 101). Facilities participating in Medicare and Medicaid programs shall comply with that code.

1.1.F.

The health care provider shall supply for each project a functional program for the facility that describes the purpose of the project, the projected demand or utilization, staffing patterns, departmental relationships, space requirements, and other basic information relating to fulfillment of the institution's objectives. This program may include a description of each function or service; the operational space required for each function; the number of staff or other occupants of the various spaces; the numbers, types, and areas (in net square feet) of all spaces; the special design features; the systems of operation; and the interrelationships of various functions and spaces. The functional program should include a description of those services necessary for the complete operation of the facility. Those services available elsewhere in the institution or community need not be duplicated in the facility. The functional program should also address the potential future expansion of essential services which may be needed to accommodate increased demand. The approved functional program shall be made available for use in the development of project design and construction documents.

1.2 Renovation

1.2.A.

Where renovation or replacement work is done within an existing facility, all new work or additions, or both, shall comply, insofar as practical, with applicable sections of these Guidelines and with appropriate parts of NFPA 101, covering New Health Care Occupancies. Where major structural elements make total compliance impractical or impossible, exceptions should be considered. This does not guarantee that an exception will be granted, but does attempt to minimize restrictions on those improvements where total compliance would not substantially improve safety, but would create an unreasonable hardship. These standards should not be construed as prohibiting a single phase of improvement. (For example, a facility may plan to replace a flammable ceiling with noncombustible material but lacks funds to do other corrective work.) However, they are not intended as an encouragement to ignore deficiencies when resources are available to correct life-threatening problems. (See Section 1.4.A.)

1.2.B.

When construction is complete, the facility shall satisfy functional requirements for the appropriate classification (general hospital, skilled nursing facility, etc.) in an environment that will provide acceptable care and safety to all occupants.

1.2.C.

In renovation projects and those making additions to existing facilities, only that portion of the total facility affected by the project shall comply with applicable sections of the Guidelines and with appropriate parts of NFPA 101 covering New Health Care Occupancies.

1.2.D.

Those existing portions of the facility which are not included in the renovation but which are essential to the functioning of the complete facility, as well as existing building areas that receive less than substantial amounts of new work shall, at a minimum, comply with that section of NFPA 101 for Existing Health Care Occupancies.

1.2.E.

Conversion to other appropriate use or replacement should be considered when cost prohibits compliance with acceptable standards.

1.2.F.

When a building is converted from one occupancy to another, it shall comply with the new occupancy requirements. For purpose of life safety, a conversion from a hospital to a nursing home or vice versa is not considered a change in occupancy.

1.2.G.

When parts of an existing facility essential to continued overall facility operation cannot comply with particular standards, those standards may be temporarily waived if patient care and safety are not jeopardized.

1.2.H.

Renovations, including new additions, shall not diminish the safety level that existed prior to the start of the work; however, safety in excess of that required for new facilities is not required.

1.2.I.

Nothing in these Guidelines shall be construed as restrictive to a facility that chooses to do work or alterations as part of a phased long-range safety improvement plan. It is emphasized that all hazards to life and safety and all areas of noncompliance with applicable codes and regulations, should be corrected as soon as possible in accordance with a plan of correction.

1.3 Design Standards for the Disabled

The Americans with Disabilities Act (ADA) became law in 1990. This law extends comprehensive civil rights protection to individuals with disabilities. Under Titles II and III of the ADA, public, private, and public service hospitals and other health care facilities will need to comply with the *Accessibility Guidelines for Buildings and Facilities* (ADAAG) for alterations and new construction. The *Uniform Federal Accessibility Standards* (UFAS) also provides criteria for the disabled. Implementation of UFAS and ADAAG for federal facilities is handled in the following ways:

- Compliance with UFAS

- Compliance with ADAAG

- Compliance with a combination of UFAS and ADAAG using the most stringent criteria

Individual federal agencies will provide direction on applicable criteria to be used for the design of federal facilities.

Also available for use in providing quality design for the disabled is the American National Standards Institute (ANSI) A117.1 *American National Standard for Accessible and Usable Buildings and Facilities.*

State and local standards for accessibility and usability may be more stringent than ADA, UFAS, or ANSI A117.1. Designers and owners, therefore, must assume responsibility for verification of all applicable requirements.

*1.4 Provisions for Disasters

In locations where there is recognized potential for hurricanes, tornadoes, flooding, earthquakes, or other regional disasters, planning and design shall consider the need to protect the life safety of all health care facility occupants and the potential need for continuing services following such a disaster.

1.4.A. Wind and Earthquake Resistant Design for New Buildings

Facilities shall be designed to meet the requirements of the building codes specified in Section 1.1.A provided these requirements are substantially equivalent to ASCE 7-93. Design shall meet the requirements of ASCE 7-93.

The following model codes and provisions are essentially equivalent to the ASCE 7-93 requirements:

1988 NEHRP Provisions
1991 ICBO Uniform Building Code
1992 Supplement to the BOCA National Building Code
1992 Amendments to the SBCC Standard Building Code

1.4.A1. For those facilities that must remain operational in the aftermath of a disaster, special design is required to protect systems and essential building services such as power, water, medical gas systems, and, in certain areas, air conditioning. In addition, special consideration must be given to the likelihood of temporary loss of externally supplied power, gas, water, and communications.

1.4.A2. The owner shall provide special inspection during construction of seismic systems described in Section A.9.1.6.2 and testing in Section A.9.1.6.3 of ASCE 7-93.

1.4.A3. Roof coverings and mechanical equipment shall be securely fastened or ballasted to the supporting roof construction and shall provide weather protection for the building at the roof. Roof covering shall be applied on clean and dry decks in accordance with the manufacturer's instructions, these Guidelines, and related references. In addition to the wind force design and construction requirements specified, particular attention shall be given to roofing, entryways, glazing, and flashing design to minimize uplift, impact damage, and other damage that could seriously impair functioning of the building. If ballast is used it shall be designed so as not to become a projectile.

1.4.B.

Flood Protection, Executive Order No. 11296, was issued to minimize financial loss from flood damage to facilities constructed with federal assistance. In accordance with that order, possible flood effects shall be considered when selecting and developing the site. Insofar as possible, new facilities shall *not* be located on designated floodplains. Where this is unavoidable, consult the Corps of Engineers regional office for the latest applicable regulations pertaining to flood insurance and protection measures that may be required.

1.4.C.

Should normal operations be disrupted, the facility shall provide adequate storage capacity for, or a functional program contingency plan to obtain, the following supplies: food, sterile supplies, pharmacy supplies, linen, and water for sanitation. Such storage capacity or plans shall be sufficient for at least four continuous days of operation.

1.5 Codes and Standards

1.5.A.

Every health care facility shall provide and maintain a safe environment for patients, personnel, and the public.

1.5.B.

References made in these Guidelines to appropriate model codes and standards do not, generally, duplicate wording of the referenced codes.

NFPA's standards, especially the NFPA 101, are the basic codes of reference; but other codes and/or standards may be included as part of these standards. In the absence of state or local requirements, the project shall comply with approved nationally recognized building codes except as modified in the latest edition of the NFPA 101 and/or herein.

Design standards for ensuring accessibility for the disabled may be based upon either ADA or UFAS, in accordance with the local authority having jurisdiction. Federally assisted construction shall comply with UFAS.

Referenced code material is contained in the issue current at the time of this publication. The latest revision of code material is usually a clarification of intent and/or general improvement in safety concepts and may be used as an explanatory document for earlier code editions. Questions of applicability should be addressed as the need occurs. The actual version of a code adopted by a jurisdiction may be different. Confirm the version adopted in a specific area with the authority having jurisdiction.

1.5.C. Equivalency

Insofar as practical, these minimum standards have been established to obtain a desired performance result. Prescriptive limitations, when given, such as exact minimum dimensions or quantities, describe a condition that is commonly recognized as a practical standard for normal operation. For example, reference to a room area is for patient, equipment, and staff activities; this avoids the need for complex descriptions of procedures for appropriate functional planning.

In all cases where specific limits are described, equivalent solutions will be acceptable if the authority having jurisdiction approves them as meeting the intent of these standards. *Nothing in this document shall be construed as restricting innovations that provide an equivalent level of performance with these standards in a manner other than that which is prescribed by this document, provided that no other safety element or system is compromised in order to establish equivalency.*

National Fire Protection Association (NFPA) document 101A is a technical standard for evaluating equivalency to certain Life Safety Code 101 requirements. The Fire Safety Evaluation System (FSES) has become widely recognized as a method for establishing a safety level equivalent to the Life Safety Code. It may be useful for evaluating *existing* facilities that will be affected by renovation. For purposes of these Guidelines, the FSES is not intended to be used for *new* construction.

1.5.D. English/Metric Measurements

Metric standards of measurement are the norm for most international commerce and are being used increasingly in health facilities in the United States. Where measurements are a part of this document, English units are given as the basic standards with metric units in parenthesis.

1.5.E. List of Referenced Codes and Standards

Codes and standards that have been referenced in whole or in part in the various sections of this document are listed below. Names and addresses of originators are also included for information. The issues available at the time of publication are used. Later issues will normally be acceptable where requirements for function and safety are not reduced; however, editions of different dates may have portions renumbered or retitled. Care must be taken to ensure that appropriate sections are used.

American National Standard/Association for Advancement of Medical Instrumentation. *Hemodialysis Systems RD5-1992.*

American National Standards Institute. Standard A17.1 (ANSI A17.1). Safety Code for Elevators and Escalators.

American Society of Civil Engineers. ASCE 7-93 (formerly ANSI A58.1), *Minimum Design Loads for Buildings and Other Structures.*

American Society of Heating, Refrigerating, and Air-Conditioning Engineers (ASHRAE). *1993 Fundamentals Handbook.*

American Society of Heating, Refrigerating, and Air-Conditioning Engineers. Standard 52-92 (ASHRAE 52.1-92), *Gravimetric and Dust Spot Procedures for Testing Air Cleaning Devices Used in General Ventilation for Removing Particulate Matter.*

American Society of Heating, Refrigerating, and Air-Conditioning Engineers. Standard 55-92 (ASHRAE 55-92), *Thermal Environmental Conditions for Human Occupancy.*

American Society of Heating, Refrigerating, and Air-Conditioning Engineers. Standard 62-89 (ASHRAE 62-89), *Ventilation for Acceptable Indoor Air Quality.*

American Society of Heating, Refrigerating, and Air-Conditioning Engineers. *1995 Applications Handbook.*

American Society of Mechanical Engineers. ASME A17.1. Safety Code for Elevators and Escalators.

American Society of Mechanical Engineers. ASME A17.3. Safety Code for Existing Elevators and Escalators.

Americans with Disabilities Act

Building Officials and Codes Administrators International, Inc. *The BOCA Basic Building Code.*

Building Officials and Codes Administrators International, Inc. *The BOCA Basic Plumbing Code.*

Centers for Disease Control and Prevention (CDC). "Guidelines for Preventing the Transmission of Mycobacterium Tuberculosis in Health Care Facilities." *Morbidity and Mortality Weekly Review* 1994:43 (No. RR-13).

Centers for Disease Control and Prevention (CDC). "Guidelines for Prevention of Nosocomial Pneumonia, 1994." *American Journal of Infection Control* (22:247-292).

Code of Federal Regulations. Title 10, parts 20 and 35, *Handling of Nuclear Materials.*

Code of Federal Regulations. Title 29, part 1910, *Employee Safety and Health.*

College of American Pathologists. *Medical Laboratory Design Manual.*

Compressed Gas Association (CGA). *Standards for Medical-Surgical Vacuum Systems in Hospitals.*

DOP Penetration Test Method. MIL STD no. 282, *Filter Units, Protective Clothing, Gas-Masking Components and Related Products: Performance Test Methods.*

General Services Administration, Department of Defense, Department of Housing and Urban Development, U.S. Postal Service. *Uniform Federal Accessibility Standards* (UFAS).

Health Education and Welfare. HEW publication no. (FDA)78-2081 (available through GPO), *Food Service Sanitation Manual.*

Hydronics Institute. *Boiler Ratings: I-B-R, Cast Iron, and SBI Steel Boilers.*

Illuminating Engineering Society of North America. *Lighting Handbook* (Vol. 2, Applications).

Illuminating Engineering Society of North America. IESNA publication CP29, *Lighting for Health Facilities.*

Illuminating Engineering Society of North America. IESNA publication RP28, *Lighting for Senior Housing.*

International Conference of Building Officials (ICBO). *Uniform Building Code.*

National Association of Plumbing-Heating-Cooling Contractors (PHCC). *National Standard Plumbing Code.*

National Bureau of Standards Interagency Report. NBSIR 81-2195, *Draft Seismic Standards for Federal Buildings Prepared by Interagency Committee on Seismic Safety in Construction* (available from NTIS as no. PB81-163842).

National Council on Radiation Protection (NCRP). *Medical X-ray and Gamma Ray Protection for Energies up to 10 MeV Equipment Design and Use.*

National Council on Radiation Protection (NCRP). *Medical X-ray and Gamma Ray Protection for Energies up to 10 MeV Structural Shielding Design and Evaluation.*

National Council on Radiation Protection (NCRP). *Radiation Protection Design Guidelines for 0.1pi29100, MeV Particle Accelerator Facilities.*

National Fire Protection Association. NFPA 20. *Centrifugal Fire Pumps.*

NFPA 70. *National Electrical Code.*

NFPA 72. *Standard for the Installation, Maintenance, and Use of Protective Signaling Systems.*

NFPA 80. *Standard for Fire Doors and Windows.*

NFPA 82. *Standard on Incinerators, Waste and Linen Handling Systems and Equipment.*

NFPA 90A. *Standard for the Installation of Air Conditioning and Ventilating Systems.*

NFPA 96. *Standard for the Installation of Equipment for the Removal of Smoke and Grease-Laden Vapors from Commercial Cooking Equipment.*

NFPA 99. *Standard for Health Care Facilities.*

NFPA 101. *Life Safety Code.*

NFPA 110. *Emergency and Standby Power Systems.*

NFPA 253. *Standard Method of Test for Critical Radiant Flux of Floor Covering Systems Using a Radiant Heat Energy Source.*

NFPA 255. *Standard Method of Test of Surface Burning Characteristics of Building Materials.*

NFPA 258. *Standard Research Test Method for Determining the Smoke Generation of Solid Materials.*

NFPA 701. *Standard Method of Fire Tests for Flame-Resistant Textiles and Films.*

NFPA 801. *Recommended Fire Protection Practice for Facilities Handling Radioactive Materials.*

Southern Building Code Congress International, Inc. *Standard Building Code.*

Underwriters Laboratories, Inc. Publication no. 181.

U.S. EPA. *Methodology for Assessing Health Risks Associated with Indirect Exposure to Combustor Emissions—International.* EPA/600/6-90/003.

U.S. EPA. *The Risk Assessment Guidelines of 1986.* EPA/600/8-87/045.

1.5.F. Availability of Codes and Standards

The codes and standards that are government publications can be ordered from the Superintendent of Documents, U.S. Government Printing Office (GPO), Washington, D.C. 20402.

Copies of nongovernment publications can be obtained at the addresses listed below.

Air Conditioning and Refrigeration Institute
1501 Wilson Boulevard
Arlington, Va. 22209

American National Standards Institute
1430 Broadway
New York, N.Y. 10018

American Society of Civil Engineers
345 East 47th Street
New York, N.Y. 10017

American Society of Heating, Refrigerating, and Air-Conditioning Engineers
1741 Tullie Circle, NE
Atlanta, Ga. 30329

Architectural and Transportation Barriers Compliance Board (ATBCB)
Office of Technical Services
330 C Street, SW
Washington, D.C. 20202

American Society for Testing and Materials (ASTM)
1916 Race Street
Philadelphia, Pa. 19103

Building Officials and Code Administrators, Inc.
4051 West Flossmoor Road
Country Club Hills, Ill. 60477

Compressed Gas Association
1235 Jefferson Davis Highway
Arlington, Va. 22202

Hydronics Institute
35 Russo Place
Berkeley Heights, N.J. 07922

Illuminating Engineering Society of North America (IESNA)
IES Publication Sales
345 East 47th Street
New York, N.Y. 10017

International Conference of Building Officials
5360 South Workman Mill Road
Whittier, Calif. 90601

National Association of Plumbing-Heating-Cooling Contractors
Box 6808
180 South Washington Street
Falls Church, Va. 22046

National Council on Radiation Protection
and Measurement
7910 Woodmont Avenue, Suite 1016
Bethesda, Md. 20814

National Fire Protection Association
1 Batterymarch Park
P.O. Box 9101
Quincy, Mass. 02269-9101

National Technical Information System (NTIS)
5285 Port Royal Road
Springfield, Va. 22161

Naval Publications and Form Center
5801 Tabor Avenue
Philadelphia, Pa. 19120
(for DOP Penetration Test Method)

Southern Building Code Congress International, Inc.
900 Montclair Road
Birmingham, Ala. 35213

Underwriters Laboratories, Inc.
333 Pfingsten Road
Northbrook, Ill. 60062

U.S. Department of Justice
Americans with Disabilities Act

2. ENERGY CONSERVATION

2.1 General

The importance of energy conservation shall be considered in all phases of facility development or renovation. Proper planning and selection of mechanical and electrical systems, as well as efficient utilization of space and climatic characteristics, can significantly reduce overall energy consumption. The quality of the health care facility environment must, however, be supportive of the occupants and functions served. Design for energy conservation shall not adversely affect patient health, safety, or accepted personal comfort levels. New and innovative systems that accommodate these considerations while preserving cost effectiveness are encouraged. Architectural elements that reduce energy consumption shall be considered part of facilities design.

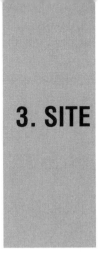

3. SITE

3.1 Location

3.1.A. Access
The site of any health care facility shall be convenient both to the community and to service vehicles, including fire protection apparatus, etc.

*3.1.B. Availability of Transportation

3.1.C. Security
Health facilities shall have security measures for patients, families, personnel, and the public consistent with the conditions and risks inherent in the location of the facility.

3.1.D. Availability of Utilities
Facilities shall be located to provide reliable utilities (water, gas, sewer, electricity). The water supply shall have the capacity to provide normal usage plus fire-fighting requirements. The electricity shall be of stable voltage and frequency.

3.2 Facility Site Design

3.2.A. Roads
Paved roads shall be provided within the property for access to all entrances and to loading and unloading docks (for delivery trucks). Hospitals with an organized emergency service shall have the emergency access well marked to facilitate entry from the public roads or streets serving the site. Other vehicular or pedestrian traffic should not conflict with access to the emergency station. In addition, access to emergency services shall be located to incur minimal damage from floods and other natural disasters. Paved walkways shall be provided for pedestrian traffic.

3.2.B. Parking
Parking shall be made available for patients, families, personnel, and the public, as described in the individual sections for specific facility types.

3.3 Environmental Pollution Control

3.3.A. Environmental Pollution
The design, construction, renovation, expansion, equipment, and operation of hospitals and medical facilities are all subject to provisions of several federal environmental pollution control laws and associated agency regulations. Moreover, many states have enacted substantially equivalent or more stringent statutes and regulations, thereby implementing national priorities under local jurisdiction while additionally incorporating local priorities (e.g., air quality related to incinerators and gas sterilizers; underground storage tanks; hazardous materials and wastes storage, handling, and disposal; storm water control; medical waste storage and disposal; and asbestos in building materials.)

The principal federal environmental statutes under which hospitals and medical facilities may be regulated include, most notably, the following:

- National Environmental Policy Act (NEPA)
- Resource Conservation and Recovery Act (RCRA)
- Superfund Amendments and Reauthorization Act (SARA)
- Clean Air Act (CAA)
- Safe Drinking Water Act (SDWA)
- Occupational Safety and Health Act (OSHA)
- Medical Waste Tracking Act (MWTA)

Consult the appropriate U.S. Department of Health and Human Services (HHS) and U.S. Environmental Protection Agency (EPA) regional offices and any other federal, state, or local authorities having jurisdiction for the latest applicable state and local regulations pertaining to environmental pollution that may affect the design, construction, or operation of the facility, including the management of industrial chemicals, pharmaceuticals, radionuclides, and wastes thereof, as well as trash, noise, and traffic (including air traffic).

Hospital and medical facilities regulated under federal, state, and local environmental pollution laws may be required to support permit applications with appropriate documentation of proposed impacts and mitigations. Such documentation is typically reported in an Environmental Impact Statement (EIS) with respect to potential impacts on the environment and in a Health Risk Assessment (HRA) with respect to potential impacts upon public health. The HRA may constitute a part or appendix of the EIS. The scope of the EIS and HRA is typically determined via consultation with appropriate regulatory agency personnel and, if required, via a "scoping" meeting at which members of the interested public are invited to express their particular concerns.

Once the EIS and/or HRA scope is established, a *Protocol* document shall be prepared for agency approval. The *Protocol* shall describe the scope and procedures to be used to conduct the assessment(s). The EIS and/or HRA shall then be prepared in accordance with a final *Protocol* approved by the appropriate agency or agencies. Approval is most likely to be obtained in a timely manner and with minimum revisions if standard methods are initially proposed for use in the EIS and/or HRA. Standard methods suitable for specific assessment tasks are set forth in particular EPA documents.

3.3.B. Equipment
Equipment should minimize the release of chlorofluorocarbons (CFCs) and any potentially toxic substances that may be used in their place. For example, the design of air conditioning systems should specify CFC alternatives and recovery systems as may be practicable.

4. EQUIPMENT

4.1 General

4.1.A.
An equipment list showing all items of equipment necessary to operate the facility shall be included in the contract documents. This list will assist in the overall coordination of the acquisition, installation, and relocation of equipment. The equipment list should include the classifications identified in Section 4.2 below and whether the items are new, existing to be relocated, owner provided, or not-in-contract.

*4.1.B.
The drawings shall indicate provisions for the installation of equipment that requires dedicated building services, or special structures, or that illustrate a major function of the space. Adjustments shall be made to the construction documents when final selections are made.

4.1.C.
Space for accessing and servicing fixed and building service equipment shall be provided.

4.1.D.
Some equipment may not be included in the construction contract but may require coordination during construction. Such equipment shall be shown in the construction documents as owner-provided or not-in-contract for purposes of coordination.

4.2 Classification

Equipment will vary to suit individual construction projects and therefore will require careful planning. Equipment to be used in projects shall be classified as building service equipment, fixed equipment, or movable equipment.

4.2.A. Building Service Equipment

Building service equipment shall include such items as heating, air conditioning, ventilation, humidification, filtration, chillers, electrical power distribution, emergency power generation, energy/utility management systems, conveying systems, and other equipment with a primary function of building service.

4.2.B. Fixed Equipment (Medical and Nonmedical)

4.2.B1. Fixed equipment includes items that are permanently affixed to the building or permanently connected to a service distribution system that is designed and installed for the specific use of the equipment. Fixed equipment may require special structural designs, electromechanical requirements, or other considerations.

a. Fixed medical equipment includes, but is not limited to, such items as fume hoods, sterilizers, communication systems, built-in casework, imaging equipment, radiotherapy equipment, lithotripters, hydrotherapy tanks, audiometry testing chambers, and lights.

b. Fixed nonmedical equipment includes, but is not limited to, items such as walk-in refrigerators, kitchen cooking equipment, serving lines, conveyors, mainframe computers, laundry, and similar equipment.

4.2.C. Movable Equipment (Medical and Nonmedical)

*4.2.C1. Movable equipment includes items that require floor space or electrical and/or mechanical connections but are portable, such as wheeled items, portable items, office-type furnishings, and monitoring equipment. Movable equipment may require special structural design, electromechanical connections, shielding, or other considerations.

a. Movable medical equipment includes, but is not limited to, portable X-ray, electroencephalogram (EEG), electrocardiogram (EKG), treadmill and exercise equipment, pulmonary function equipment, operating tables, laboratory centrifuges, examination and treatment tables, and similar equipment.

b. Movable nonmedical equipment includes, but is not limited to, personal computer stations, patient room furnishings, food service trucks, case carts and distribution carts, and other portable equipment.

*4.3 Major Technical Equipment

Major technical equipment is specialized equipment (medical or nonmedical) that is customarily installed by the manufacturer or vendor. Since major technical equipment may require special structural designs, electromechanical requirements, or other considerations, close coordination between owner, building designer, installer, construction contractors, and others is required.

4.4 Equipment Shown on Drawings

Equipment which is not included in the construction contract but which requires mechanical or electrical service connections or construction modifications shall, insofar as practical, be identified on the design development documents to provide coordination with the architectural, mechanical, and electrical phases of construction.

4.5 Electronic Equipment

Special consideration shall be given to protecting computerized equipment such as multiphasic laboratory testing units, as well as computers, from power surges and spikes that might damage the equipment or programs. Consideration shall also be given to the addition of a constant power source where loss of data input might compromise patient care.

5. CONSTRUCTION

*5.1 Planning and Design

Continual health care facility upgrade through renovation and new construction of hospital facilities can create conditions which can be hazardous to patients. Design and planning for such projects in the health care facilities shall require consultation from infection control professionals and safety personnel. Early involvement in the conceptual phase will help ascertain the risk assessment for susceptible patient location and disruption of essential patient services. Control for clean to dirty airflow, interruption of utility and/or building/equipment services, and communication requirements shall be specified in the project bid documents in order to ensure construction specification compliance.

*5.2 Phasing

Projects involving renovation of existing buildings shall include phasing to minimize disruption of existing patient services. This phasing is essential to ensure a safe environment in patient care areas. Phasing will include assurance for clean to dirty airflow, emergency procedures, criteria for interruption of protection, construction of roof surfaces, written notification of interruptions, and communication authority. The effects of noise and vibration will affect patients, and procedures must be planned for accordingly. The renovation areas shall be isolated from the occupied areas during construction using airtight barriers, and exhaust airflow shall be sufficient to maintain negative air pressure in the construction zone. Air quality requirements shall be maintained as described in Tables 2 and 6.

5.3 Commissioning

Acceptance criteria for mechanical systems shall be specified. Crucial ventilation specifications for air balance and filtration shall be verified before Owner acceptance. Areas requiring special ventilation include surgical services, protective environments, airborne infection isolation rooms, laboratories, and local exhaust systems for hazardous agents. These areas shall be recognized as requiring mechanical systems that ensure infection control, and ventilation deficiencies shall not be accepted. Acceptance criteria for local exhaust systems dealing with hazardous agents shall be specified and verified.

5.4 Nonconforming Conditions

It is not always financially feasible to renovate the entire existing structure in accordance with these Guidelines. In such cases, authorities having jurisdiction may grant approval to renovate portions of the structure if facility operation and patient safety in the renovated areas are not jeopardized by the existing features of sections retained without complete corrective measures.

6. RECORD DRAWINGS AND MANUALS

6.1 Drawings

Upon occupancy of the building or portion thereof, the owner shall be provided with a complete set of legible drawings showing construction, fixed equipment, and mechanical and electrical systems, as installed or built. Drawings shall include a fire protection plan for each floor reflecting NFPA 101 requirements.

6.2 Equipment Manuals

Upon completion of the contract, the owner shall be furnished with a complete set of manufacturers' operating, maintenance, and preventive maintenance instructions; parts lists; and procurement information with numbers and a description for each piece of equipment. Operating staff shall also be provided with instructions on how to properly operate systems and equipment. Required information shall include energy ratings as needed for future conservation calculations.

6.3 Design Data

The owners shall be provided with complete design data for the facility. This shall include structural design loadings; summary of heat loss assumption and calculations; estimated water consumption; medical gas outlet listing; list of applicable codes; and electric power requirements of installed equipment. All such data shall be supplied to facilitate future alterations, additions, and changes, including, but not limited to, energy audits and retrofit for energy conservation.

7. GENERAL HOSPITAL

7.1 General Considerations

7.1.A. Functions
There shall be for each project a functional program for the facility in accordance with Section 1.1.F.

7.1.B. Standards
The general hospital shall meet all the standards described herein. Deviations shall be described and justified in the functional program for specific approval by the authorities having jurisdiction.

7.1.C. Sizes
Department size and clear floor areas will depend upon program requirements and organization of services within the hospital. Some functions may be combined or shared providing the layout does not compromise safety standards and medical and nursing practices.

7.1.D. Parking
Each new facility, major addition, or major change in function shall have parking space to satisfy the needs of patients, personnel, and public. *A formal parking study is desirable.* In the absence of such a study, provide one space for each bed plus one space for each employee normally present on any single weekday shift. This ratio may be reduced in an area convenient to public transportation or public parking facilities, or where carpool or other arrangements to reduce traffic have been developed. Additional parking may be required to accommodate outpatient and other services. Separate and additional space shall be provided for service delivery vehicles and vehicles utilized for emergency patients.

*7.1.E. Swing Beds
When the concept of swing beds is part of the functional program, care shall be taken to include requirements for all intended categories.

7.2 Nursing Unit (Medical and Surgical)

See other sections of this document for special-care area units such as recovery rooms, critical care units, pediatric units, rehabilitation units, and skilled nursing care or other specialty units.

Each nursing unit shall include the following (see Section 1.2 for waiver of standards where existing conditions make absolute compliance impractical):

7.2.A. Patient Rooms
Each patient room shall meet the following standards:

7.2.A1. Maximum room capacity shall be two patients. Where renovation work is undertaken and the present capacity is more than two patients, maximum room capacity shall be no more than the present capacity with a maximum of four patients.

*7.2.A2. In new construction, patient rooms shall have a minimum of 100 square feet (9.29 square meters) of clear floor area per bed in multiple-bed rooms and 120 square feet (11.15 square meters) of clear floor area for single-bed rooms, exclusive of toilet rooms, closets, lockers, wardrobes, alcoves, or vestibules. The dimensions and arrangement of rooms shall be such that there is a minimum of 3 feet (0.91 meter) between the sides and foot of the bed and any wall or any other fixed obstruction. In multiple-bed rooms, a clearance of 4 feet (1.22 meters) shall be available at the foot of each bed to permit the passage of equipment and beds. Minor encroachments, including columns and lavatories, that do not interfere with functions may be ignored when determining space requirements for patient rooms. Where renovation work is undertaken, every effort shall be made to meet the above minimum standards. If it is not possible to meet the above square-foot standards, the authorities having jurisdiction may grant approval to deviate from this requirement. In such cases, patient rooms shall have no less than 80 square feet (7.43 square meters) of clear floor area per bed in multiple-bed areas and 100 square feet (9.29 square meters) of clear floor area in single-bed rooms.

*7.2.A3. Each patient room shall have a window in accordance with Section 7.28.A10.

*7.2.A4. Handwashing facilities shall be provided to serve each patient room. These handwashing facilities shall be located in the toilet room.

7.2.A5. Each patient shall have access to a toilet room without having to enter the general corridor area. One toilet room shall serve no more than four beds and no more than two patient rooms. In new construction, an additional handwashing facility shall be placed in the patient room where the toilet room serves more than two beds. The toilet room shall contain a water closet and a handwashing facility and the door shall swing outward or be double acting.

7.2.A6. Each patient shall have within his or her room a separate wardrobe, locker, or closet suitable for hanging full-length garments and for storing personal effects.

7.2.A7. In multiple-bed rooms, visual privacy from casual observation by other patients and visitors shall be provided for each patient. The design for privacy shall not restrict patient access to the entrance, lavatory, or toilet.

7.2.B. Service Areas
Provision for the services listed below shall be in or readily available to each nursing unit. The size and location of each service area will depend upon the numbers and types of beds served. Identifiable spaces are required for each of the indicated functions. Each service area may be arranged and located to serve more than one nursing unit but, unless noted otherwise, at least one such service area shall be provided on each nursing floor. Where the words *room* or *office* are used, a separate, enclosed space for the one named function is intended; otherwise, the described area may be a specific space in another room or common area.

7.2.B1. Administrative center or nurse station. This area shall have space for counters and storage and shall have convenient access to handwashing facilities. It may be combined with or include centers for reception and communication. Preferably, the station should permit visual observation of all traffic into the unit.

7.2.B2. Dictation area. This area should be adjacent to but separate from the nurse station.

7.2.B3. Nurse or supervisor office.

7.2.B4. Handwashing fixtures, conveniently accessible to the nurse station, medication station, and nourishment center. One handwashing fixture may serve several areas if convenient to each.

7.2.B5. Charting facilities.

7.2.B6. Toilet room(s) conveniently located for staff use (may be unisex).

7.2.B7. Staff lounge facilities shall be provided. These facilities may be on another floor.

7.2.B8. Securable closets or cabinet compartments for the personal articles of nursing personnel, located in or near the nurse station. At a minimum, these shall be large enough for purses and billfolds. Coats may be stored in closets or cabinets on each floor or in a central staff locker area.

7.2.B9. Multipurpose room(s) for staff, patients, patients' families for patient conferences, reports, education, training sessions, and consultation. These rooms must be accessible to each nursing unit. They may be on other floors if convenient for regular use. One such room may serve several nursing units and/or departments.

7.2.B10. Examination/treatment room(s). Such rooms may be omitted if all patient rooms in the nursing unit are single-bed rooms. Centrally located examination and treatment room(s) may serve more than one nursing unit on the same floor. Such rooms shall have a minimum floor area of 120 square feet (11.15 square meters). The room shall contain a handwashing fixture; storage facilities; and a desk, counter, or shelf space for writing.

7.2.B11. Clean workroom or clean supply room. If the room is used for preparing patient care items, it shall contain a work counter, a handwashing fixture, and storage facilities for clean and sterile supplies. If the room is used only for storage and holding as part of a system for distribution of clean and sterile materials, the work counter and handwashing fixture may be omitted. Soiled and clean workrooms or holding rooms shall be separated and have no direct connection.

7.2.B12. Soiled workroom or soiled holding room. This room shall be separate from the clean workroom. The soiled workroom shall contain a clinical sink (or equivalent flushing-rim fixture). The room shall contain a lavatory (or handwashing fixture). The above fixtures shall both have a hot and cold mixing faucet. The room shall have a work counter and space for separate covered containers for soiled linen and waste. Rooms used only for temporary holding of soiled material may omit the clinical sink and work counter. If the flushing-rim clinical sink is eliminated, facilities for cleaning bedpans shall be provided elsewhere.

7.2.B13. Medication station. Provision shall be made for distribution of medications. This may be done from a medicine preparation room or unit, from a self-contained medicine dispensing unit, or by another approved system.

a. Medicine preparation room. This room shall be under visual control of the nursing staff. It shall contain a work counter, a sink adequate for handwashing, refrigerator, and locked storage for controlled drugs. When a medicine preparation room is to be used to store one or more self-contained medicine dispensing units, the room shall be designed with adequate space to prepare medicines with the self-contained medicine dispensing unit(s) present.

b. Self-contained medicine dispensing unit. A self-contained medicine dispensing unit may be located at the nurse station, in the clean workroom, or in an alcove, provided the unit has adequate security for controlled drugs and adequate lighting to easily identify drugs. Convenient access to handwashing facilities shall be provided. (Standard cup-sinks provided in many self-contained units are not adequate for handwashing.)

7.2.B14. Clean linen storage. Each nursing unit shall contain a designated area for clean linen storage. This may be within the clean workroom, a separate closet, or an approved distribution system on each floor. If a closed cart system is used, storage may be in an alcove. It must be out of the path of normal traffic and under staff control.

7.2.B15. Nourishment station. There shall be a nourishment station with sink, work counter, refrigerator, storage cabinets, and equipment for hot and cold nourishments between scheduled meals. The nourishment station shall include space for trays and dishes used for nonscheduled meal service. Provisions and space shall be included for separate temporary storage of unused and soiled dietary trays not picked up at meal time. Handwashing facilities shall be in or immediately accessible from the nourishment station.

7.2.B16. Ice machine. Each nursing unit shall have equipment to provide ice for treatments and nourishment. Ice-making equipment may be in the clean work room/holding room or at the nourishment station. Ice intended for human consumption shall be from self-dispensing ice makers.

7.2.B17. Equipment storage room or alcove. Appropriate room(s) or alcove(s) shall be provided for storage of equipment necessary for patient care and as required by the functional program. This room may serve more than one unit on the same floor. Its location shall not interfere with the flow of traffic.

7.2.B18. Storage space for stretchers and wheelchairs shall be provided in a strategic location, without restricting normal traffic.

7.2.B19. Showers and bathtubs. When individual bathing facilities are not provided in patient rooms, there shall be at least one shower and/or bathtub for each 12 beds without such facilities. Each bathtub or shower shall be in an individual room or enclosure that provides privacy for bathing, drying, and dressing. Special bathing facilities, including space for attendant, shall be provided for patients on stretchers, carts, and wheelchairs at the ratio of one per 100 beds or a fraction thereof. This may be on a separate floor if convenient for use.

7.2.B20. Patient toilet room(s), in addition to those serving bed areas, shall be conveniently located to multipurpose room(s) and to each central bathing facility. Patient toilet rooms serving multipurpose rooms may also be designated for public use.

7.2.B21. Emergency equipment storage. Space shall be provided for emergency equipment that is under direct control of the nursing staff, such as a cardiopulmonary resuscitation (CPR) cart. This space shall be located in an area appropriate to the functional program, but out of normal traffic.

7.2.B22. Housekeeping room. One housekeeping room shall be provided for each nursing unit or nursing floor. It shall be directly accessible from the unit or floor and may serve more than one nursing unit on a floor. At least one housekeeping room per floor shall contain a service sink or floor receptor and provisions for storage of supplies and housekeeping equipment.

Note: This housekeeping room may not be used for other departments and nursing units that require separate housekeeping rooms.

7.2.C. Airborne Infection Isolation Room(s)
Note: The airborne infection isolation room requirements contained in these Guidelines for particular service areas throughout a facility should be predicated on an "infection control risk assessment" and based on the needs of specific community and patient populations served by an individual organization. The number of airborne infection isolation rooms for individual patient units shall be increased based upon an "infection control risk assessment" or by a multidisciplinary group designated for that purpose. This process ensures a more accurate determination of environmentally safe and appropriate room types and spatial needs. It is suggested that reference be made to the Center for Disease Control and Prevention (CDC) "Guidelines for Preventing the Transmission of Mycobacterium Tuberculosis in Health Care Facilities" as they appear in the *Federal Register* dated October 28, 1994 and the *Morbidity and Mortality Weekly Report (MMWR)* 1994:43(No. RR-13), and the "Guidelines for Prevention of Nosocomial Pneumonia, 1994," published by CDC in the *American Journal of Infection Control* (22:247-292).

7.2.C1. At least one airborne infection isolation room shall be provided. These rooms may be located within individual nursing units and used for normal acute care when not required for isolation cases, or they may be grouped as a separate isolation unit. Each room shall contain only one bed and shall comply with the acute-care patient room section of this document as well as the following:

7.2.C2. Each airborne infection isolation room shall have an area for handwashing, gowning, and storage of clean and soiled materials located directly outside or immediately inside the entry door to the room.

7.2.C3. Airborne infection isolation room perimeter walls, ceiling, and floors, including penetrations, shall be sealed tightly so that air does not infiltrate the environment from the outside or from other spaces.

7.2.C4. Airborne infection isolation room(s) shall have self-closing devices on all room exit doors.

7.2.C5. Separate toilet, bathtub (or shower), and handwashing facilities are required for each airborne infection isolation room.

7.2.C6. Airborne infection isolation rooms may be used for noninfectious patients when not needed for patients with airborne infectious disease.

*7.2.D. Protective Environment Room(s)
Note: The differentiating factor between protective environment rooms and other patient rooms is the requirement for positive air pressure relative to adjoining spaces with all supply air passing through HEPA filters with 99.97 percent efficiency for particles >3 micron μm in size. When determined by an infection control risk assessment, special design considerations and air ventilation to ensure the protection of patients with these conditions shall be required. The appropriate numbers and location of protective environment rooms shall be concluded by the infection control risk assessment. Protective environment room(s) shall contain only one bed and comply with Section 7.2.C. Special ventilation requirements are found in Table 2. Also see special guidelines for protective environment rooms during renovation and construction in Section 5.1.

As designated by the functional program, both airborne infection isolation and protective environment rooms may be required. Many facilities care for patients with an extreme susceptibility to infection, e.g., immunosuppressed patients with prolonged granulocytopenia, most notably bone marrow recipients; or solid-organ transplant recipients and patients with hematological malignancies who are receiving chemotherapy and are severely granulocytopenic. These rooms are not intended for use with patients diagnosed with HIV infection or AIDS, unless they are also severely granulocytopenic. Generally, protective environments are not needed in community hospitals, unless these facilities take care of these types of patients. The appropriate clinical staff should be consulted regarding room type and spatial needs to meet facility infection control requirements should be incorporated in design programming.

7.2.E. Seclusion Room(s)
The hospital shall provide one or more single bedrooms for patients needing close supervision for medical and/or psychiatric care. This may be part of the psychiatric unit described in Section 7.6. If the single bedroom(s) is part of the acute-care nursing unit, the provisions of Section 7.6.A shall apply, with the following exceptions: each room shall be for single occupancy; each shall be located to permit staff observation of the entrance, preferably adjacent to the nurse station; and each shall be designed to minimize the potential for escape, hiding, injury, or suicide. If vision panels are used for observation of patients, the arrangement shall insure patient privacy and prevent casual observation by visitors and other patients.

7.3 Critical Care Units

The critical care units require special space and equipment considerations for effective staff functions. In addition, space arrangement shall include provisions for immediate access of emergency equipment from other departments.

Not every hospital will provide all types of critical care. Some hospitals may have a small combined unit; others may have separate, sophisticated units for highly specialized treatments. Critical care units shall comply in size, number, and type with these standards and with the functional program. The following standards are intended for the more common types of critical care services and shall be appropriate to needs defined in functional programs. Where specialized services are required, additions and/or modifications shall be made as necessary for efficient, safe, and effective patient care.

7.3.A. Critical Care (General)

The following shall apply to all types of critical care units unless otherwise noted. Each unit shall comply with the following provisions:

7.3.A1. The location shall offer convenient access from the emergency, respiratory therapy, laboratory, radiology, surgery, and other essential departments and services as defined by the functional program. It shall be located so that the medical emergency resuscitation teams may be able to respond promptly to emergency calls within minimum travel time. The location shall be arranged to eliminate the need for through traffic.

*7.3.A2. In new construction, where elevator transport is required for critically ill patients, the size of the cab and mechanisms and controls shall meet the specialized needs.

*7.3.A3. In new construction, each patient space (whether separate rooms, cubicles, or multiple bed space) shall have a minimum of 150 square feet (13.94 square meters) of clear floor area with a minimum headwall width of 12 feet (3.66 meters) per bed, exclusive of anterooms, vestibules, toilet rooms, closets, lockers, wardrobes, and/or alcoves.

In renovation of existing intensive care units, every effort shall be made to meet the above minimum standards. If it is not possible to meet the above square-foot standards, the authorities having jurisdiction may grant approval to deviate from this requirement. In such cases, separate rooms or cubicles for single patient use shall be no less than 130 square feet (12.09 square meters) and multiple bed space shall contain at least 110 square feet (10.23 square meters) per bed.

7.3.A4. When private rooms or cubicles are provided, view panels to the corridor shall be required and shall have drapes or curtains which may be closed. Where only one door is provided to a bed space, it shall be at least 4 feet (1.22 meters) wide and arranged to minimize interference with movement of beds and large equipment. Sliding doors shall not have floor tracks and shall have hardware that minimizes jamming possibilities. Where sliding doors are used for access to cubicles within a suite, a 3-foot-wide (.91 meters) swinging door may also be provided for personnel communication.

7.3.A5. Each patient bed area shall have space at each bedside for visitors, and provisions for visual privacy from casual observation by other patients and visitors. For both adult and pediatric units, there shall be a minimum of 8 feet (2.44 meters) between beds.

7.3.A6. Each patient bed shall have visual access, other than skylights, to the outside environment with not less than one outside window in each patient bed area. In renovation projects, clerestory windows with windowsills above the heights of adjacent ceilings may be used, provided they afford patients a view of the exterior and are equipped with appropriate forms of glare and sun control. Distance from the patient bed to the outside window shall not exceed 50 feet (15.24 meters). When partitioned cubicles are used, patients' view to outside windows may be through no more than two separate clear vision panels.

7.3.A7. Systems for rapid and easy information exchange with a hospital are important. Nurse calling systems for two-way voice communication shall be provided in accordance with Section 7.32.G. The call system for the unit shall include provisions for an emergency code resuscitation alarm to summon assistance from outside the critical care unit.

7.3.A8. Handwashing fixtures shall be convenient to nurse stations and patient bed areas. There shall be at least one handwashing fixture for every three beds in open plan areas, and one in each patient room. The handwashing fixture should be located near the entrance to the patient cubicle or room, should be sized to minimize splashing water onto the floor, and should be equipped with hands-free operable controls.

*7.3.A9. Administrative center or nurse station. This area shall have space for counters and storage. It may be combined with or include centers for reception and communication. There shall be direct or remote visual observation between the administration center or nurse station and all patient beds in the critical care unit.

7.3.A10. Each unit shall contain equipment for continuous monitoring, with visual displays for each patient at the bedside and at the nurse station. Monitors shall be located to permit easy viewing and access but not interfere with access to the patient.

7.3.A11. Emergency equipment storage. Space that is easily accessible to the staff shall be provided for emergency equipment such as a CPR cart.

*7.3.A12. Medication station. Provision shall be made for storage and distribution of emergency drugs and routine medications. This may be done from a medicine preparation room or unit, from a self-contained medicine dispensing unit, or by another system. If used, a medicine preparation room or unit shall be under visual control of nursing staff. It shall contain a work counter, cabinets for storage of supplies, sink with hot and cold water supply, refrigerator for pharmaceuticals, and doubled locked storage for controlled substances. Convenient access to handwashing facilities shall be provided. (Standard cup-sinks provided in many self-contained units are not adequate for handwashing.)

7.3.A13. The electrical, medical gas, heating, and air conditioning shall support the needs of the patients and critical care team members under normal and emergency situations.

7.3.A14. At least one airborne infection isolation room shall be provided. The number of airborne infection isolation rooms shall be determined based on an infection control risk assessment. Each room shall contain only one bed and shall comply with the requirements of Section 7.2.C. Special ventilation requirements are found in Table 2.

*7.3.A15. The following additional service spaces shall be immediately available within each critical care suite. These may be shared by more than one critical care unit provided that direct access is available from each.

a. Securable closets or cabinet compartments for the personal effects of nursing personnel, located in or near the nurse station. At a minimum, these shall be large enough for purses and billfolds. Coats may be stored in closets or cabinets on each floor or in a central staff locker area.

b. Clean workroom or clean supply room. If the room is used for preparing patient care items, it shall contain a work counter, a handwashing fixture, and storage facilities for clean and sterile supplies. If the room is used only for storage and holding as part of a system for distribution of clean and sterile supply materials, the work counter and handwashing fixture may be omitted. Soiled and clean workrooms or holding rooms shall be separated and have no direct connection.

c. Clean linen storage. There shall be a designated area for clean linen storage. This may be within the clean workroom, a separate closet, or an approved distribution system on each floor. If a closed cart system is used, storage may be in an alcove. It must be out of the path of normal traffic and under staff control.

d. Soiled workroom or soiled holding room. This room shall be separate from the clean workroom. The soiled workroom shall contain a clinical sink (or equivalent flushing-rim fixture). The room shall contain a lavatory (or handwashing fixture). The above fixtures shall have a hot and cold mixing faucet. The room shall have a work counter and space for separate covered containers for soiled linen and a variety of waste types. Rooms used only for temporary holding of soiled material may omit the clinical sink and work counter. If the flushing-rim clinical sink is eliminated, facilities for cleaning bedpans shall be provided elsewhere.

e. Nourishment station. There shall be a nourishment station with sink, work counter, refrigerator, storage cabinets, and equipment for hot and cold nourishments between scheduled meals. The nourishment station shall include space for trays and dishes used for nonscheduled meal service. Provisions and space shall be included for separate temporary storage of unused and soiled dietary trays not picked up at meal time. Handwashing facilities shall be in or immediately accessible from the nourishment station.

f. Ice machine. There shall be available equipment to provide ice for treatments and nourishment. Ice-making equipment may be in the clean work room or at the nourishment station. Ice intended for human consumption shall be from self-dispensing ice makers.

*g. Equipment storage room or alcove. Appropriate room(s) or alcove(s) shall be provided for storage of large items of equipment necessary for patient care and as required by the functional program. Its location shall not interfere with the flow of traffic.

h. An X-ray viewing facility shall be in the unit.

7.3.A16. The following shall be provided and may be located outside the unit if conveniently accessible.

a. A visitors' waiting room will be provided with convenient access to telephones and toilets. One waiting room may serve several critical care units.

b. Adequate office space immediately adjacent to the critical care unit will be available for critical care medical and nursing management/administrative personnel. The offices should be large enough to permit consulting with members of the critical care team and visitors. The offices will be linked with the unit by telephone or an intercommunications system.

c. Staff lounge(s) and toilet(s) shall be located so that staff may be recalled quickly to the patient area in emergencies. The lounge shall have telephone or intercom and emergency code alarm connections to the critical care unit it serves. If not provided elsewhere, provision for the storage of coats, etc., shall be made in this area. Consideration should be given to providing adequate furnishings, equipment, and space for comfortable seating and the preparation and consumption of snacks and beverages. One lounge may serve adjacent critical care areas.

d. A special procedures room shall be provided if required by the functional program.

e. Sleeping and personal care accommodations for staff on 24-hour, on-call work schedules.

f. Multipurpose room(s) for staff, patients, and patients' families for patient conferences, reports, education, training sessions, and consultation. These rooms must be accessible to each nursing unit.

g. A housekeeping room shall be provided within or immediately adjacent to the critical care unit. It shall not be shared with other nursing units or departments. It shall contain a service sink or floor receptor and provisions for storage of supplies and housekeeping equipment.

h. Storage space for stretchers and wheelchairs shall be provided in a strategic location, without restricting normal traffic.

i. Laboratory, radiology, respiratory therapy, and pharmacy services shall be available. These services may be provided from the central departments or from satellite facilities as required by the functional program.

7.3.B. Coronary Critical Care Unit

Coronary patients have special needs. They are often fully aware of their surroundings but still need immediate and critical emergency care. In addition to the standards set forth in Section 7.3.A, the following standards apply to the coronary critical care unit:

7.3.B1. Each coronary patient shall have a separate room for acoustical and visual privacy.

7.3.B2. Each coronary patient shall have access to a toilet in the room. (Portable commodes may be used in lieu of individual toilets, but provisions must be made for their storage, servicing, and odor control.)

7.3.C. Combined Medical/Surgical and Coronary Critical Care

If medical, surgical, and coronary critical care services are combined in one critical care unit, at least 50 percent of the beds must be located in private rooms or cubicles. (Note: Medical/surgical patients may utilize open areas or private rooms as needed and available but, insofar as possible, coronary patients should not be accommodated in open ward areas.)

7.3.D. Pediatric Critical Care

Critically ill pediatric patients have unique physical and psychological needs. Not every hospital can or should attempt to have a separate pediatric critical care unit. Many hospitals will be able to safely transfer their patients to other facilities offering appropriate services. If a facility has a specific pediatric critical care unit, the functional program must include consideration for staffing, isolation, and the safe transportation of critically ill pediatric patients, along with life support and environmental systems, from other areas. At least one airborne infection control room shall be provided, with provisions for observation of the patient. The total number of infection control rooms shall be increased based upon an infection control risk assessment. All room(s) shall comply with the requirements of Section 7.2.C.

In addition to the standards previously listed for critical care units, each pediatric critical care unit shall include:

7.3.D1. Space at each bedside for parents.

*7.3.D2. Sleeping space for parents who may be required to spend long hours with the patient. If the sleeping area is separate from the patient area, it must be in communication with the critical care unit staff.

7.3.D3. Consultation/demonstration room within, or convenient to, the pediatric critical care unit for private discussions.

7.3.D4. Provisions for formula storage. These may be outside the pediatric critical care unit but must be available for use at all times.

7.3.D5. Separate storage cabinets or closets for toys and games for use by the pediatric patients.

7.3.D6. Additional storage for cots, bed linens, and other items needed to accommodate parents overnight.

*7.3.D7. Space allowance.

7.3.D8. Examination and treatment room(s). Centrally located examination and treatment room(s) may serve more than one floor and/or nursing unit. Examination and treatment rooms shall have a minimum floor area of 120 square feet (11.15 square meters). The room shall contain a handwashing fixture; storage facilities; and a desk, counter, or shelf space for writing.

7.3.E. Newborn Intensive Care Units

Each Newborn Intensive Care Unit (NICU) shall include or comply with the following:

7.3.E1. The NICU shall have a clearly identified entrance and reception area for families. The area shall permit visual observation and contact with all traffic entering the unit. A scrub area shall be provided at each public entrance to the patient care area(s) of the NICU. All sinks shall be hands-free operable and large enough to contain splashing.

7.3.E2. At least one door to each room in the unit must be large enough to accommodate portable X-ray equipment. A door 44 inches (111.76 centimeters) wide should accommodate most X-ray equipment. Both width and height must be considered.

7.3.E3. There should be efficient and controlled access to the unit from the Labor and Delivery area, the Emergency Room, or other referral entry points.

7.3.E4. When viewing windows are provided, provision shall be made to control casual viewing of infants.

7.3.E5. In the interest of noise control, sound attenuation shall be a design factor.

*7.3.E6. Provisions shall be made for indirect lighting and high-intensity lighting in all nurseries.

7.3.E7. A central area shall serve as a control station, shall have space for counters and storage, and shall have convenient access to handwashing facilities. It may be combined with or include centers for reception and communication and patient monitoring.

7.3.E8. Each patient care space shall contain a minimum of 100 square feet (9.29 square meters) excluding sinks and aisles. There shall be an aisle for circulation adjacent to each patient care space with a minimum width of 3 feet (0.91 meter).

7.3.E9. An airborne infection isolation room is required in at least one level of nursery care. The room shall be enclosed and separated from the nursery unit with provisions for observation of the infant from adjacent nurseries or control area(s). All airborne infection isolation rooms shall comply with the requirements of Section 7.2.C, except for separate toilet, bathtub, or shower.

7.3.E10. Blood gas lab facilities should be immediately accessible.

7.3.E11. Physician's sleeping facilities with access to a toilet and shower shall be provided. If not contained within the unit itself, the area shall have a telephone or intercom connection to the patient care area.

*7.3.E12. Sleeping space may be needed for parents who may be required to spend long hours with the neonate. This space may be separate from the unit, but must be in communication with the Newborn Critical Care Unit staff.

7.3.E13. A respiratory therapy work area and storage room shall be provided.

7.3.E14. A consultation/demonstration/breast feeding or pump room shall be provided convenient to the unit. Provision shall be made, either within the room or conveniently located nearby, for sink, counter, refrigeration and freezing, storage for pump and attachments, and educational materials.

7.3.E15. Provide charting and dictation space for physicians.

7.3.E16. Medication station. See Section 7.3.A12.

*7.3.E17. Clean workroom or clean supply room. See Section 7.3.A.15b.

7.3.E18. Soiled workroom or soiled holding room. See Section 7.3.A.15d

7.3.E19. Provide a lounge, locker room, and staff toilet within or adjacent to the unit suite for staff use.

7.3.E20. Emergency equipment storage. Space shall be provided for emergency equipment that is under direct control of the nursing staff, such as a CPR cart. This space shall be located in an area appropriate to the functional program, but out of normal traffic.

7.3.E21. Housekeeping room. One housekeeping room shall be provided for the unit. It shall be directly accessible from the unit and be dedicated for the exclusive use of the neonatal critical care unit. It shall contain a service sink or floor receptor and provisions for storage of supplies and housekeeping equipment.

7.3.E22. Space should be provided for the following:

a. A visitors' waiting room. See Section 7.3.A.16a.

b. Nurses/supervisors office or station. See Section 7.3.A.16b.

c. Multipurpose room(s) for staff, patients and patients' families for patient conferences, reports, education, training sessions, and consultation. These rooms must be accessible to each nursing unit. They may be on other floors if convenient for regular use. One such room may serve several nursing units and/or departments.

*7.4 Newborn Nurseries

Hospitals having 25 or more postpartum beds shall have a separate nursery that provides continuing care for infants requiring close observation (for example, those with low birth weight). The minimum floor area per infant shall be 50 square feet (4.65 square meters), exclusive of auxiliary work areas, with provisions for at least 4 feet (1.22 meters) between and at all sides of bassinets.

Note: Normal newborn infants shall be housed in nurseries that comply with the standards below. Location shall be convenient to the postpartum nursing unit and obstetrical facilities. The nurseries shall be located and arranged to preclude the need for nonrelated pedestrian traffic. No nursery shall open directly into another nursery. See Section 7.5 for pediatric nurseries. See Section 7.3.E for critical care units for neonatal infants.

7.4.A. General
Each nursery shall contain:

7.4.A1. At least one lavatory, equipped with handwashing controls that can be operated without use of hands, for each eight infant stations.

7.4.A2. Glazed observation windows to permit the viewing of infants from public areas, workrooms, and adjacent nurseries.

7.4.A3. Convenient, accessible storage for linens and infant supplies at each nursery room.

7.4.A4. A consultation/demonstration/breast feeding or pump room shall be provided convenient to the nursery. Provision shall be made, either within the room or conveniently located nearby, for sink, counter, refrigeration and freezing, storage for pump and attachments, and educational materials. The area provided for the unit for these purposes, when conveniently located, may be shared by the newborn nursery.

7.4.A5. Enough space shall be provided for parents to stay 24 hours.

7.4.A6. An airborne infection isolation room is required in or near at least one level of nursery care. The room shall be enclosed and separated from the nursery unit with provisions for observation of the infant from adjacent nurseries or control area(s). All airborne infection isolation rooms shall comply with the requirements of Section 7.2.C, except for separate toilet, bathtub, or shower.

7.4.B. Full-Term Nursery
Each full-term nursery room shall contain no more than 16 infant stations. The minimum floor area shall be 24 square feet (2.23 square meters) for each infant station, exclusive of auxiliary work areas. When a rooming-in program is used, the total number of bassinets provided in these units may be appropriately reduced, but the full-term nursery may not be omitted in its entirety from any facility that includes delivery services. (When facilities use a rooming-in program in which all infants are returned to the nursery at night, a reduction in nursery size may not be practical.)

7.4.B1. Baby Holding Nurseries
Hospitals may replace traditional nurseries with baby holding nurseries in postpartum and labor-delivery-recovery-postpartum (LDRP) units. The minimum floor area per bassinet, ventilation, electrical, and medical vacuum and gases shall be the same as that required for a full-term nursery. These holding nurseries should be next to the nurse station on these units. The holding nursery shall be sized to accommodate the percentage of newborns who do not remain with their mothers during the postpartum stay.

7.4.C. Charting Facilities
Provision shall be made for physician and nurse charting and dictation. This may be in a separate room or part of the workroom.

*7.4.D. Workroom(s)
Each nursery room shall be served by a connecting workroom. The workroom shall contain scrubbing and gowning facilities at the entrance for staff and housekeeping personnel, work counter, refrigerator, storage for supplies, and handwashing fixture. One workroom may serve more than one nursery room provided that required services are convenient to each.

The workroom serving the full-term and continuing care nurseries may be omitted if equivalent work and storage areas and facilities, including those for scrubbing and gowning, are provided within that nursery. Space required for work areas located within the nursery is in addition to the area required for infant care.

Adequate provision shall be made for storage of emergency cart(s) and equipment out of traffic and for the sanitary storage and disposal of soiled waste.

7.4.E. Infant Examination and Treatment Areas
Such areas, when required by the functional program, shall contain a work counter, storage facilities, and a handwashing fixture.

7.4.F. Infant Formula Facilities

7.4.F1. When infant formula is prepared on-site, direct access from the formula preparation room to any nursery room is prohibited. The room may be located near the nursery or at other appropriate locations in the hospital, but must include:

a. Cleanup facilities for washing and sterilizing supplies. This area shall include a handwashing fixture, facilities for bottle washing, a work counter, and sterilization equipment.

b. Separate room for preparing infant formula. This room shall contain warming facilities, refrigerator, work counter, formula sterilizer, storage facilities, and a handwashing fixture.

c. Refrigerated storage and warming facilities for infant formula accessible for use by nursery personnel at all times.

7.4.F2. If a commercial infant formula is used, the separate clean-up and preparation rooms may be omitted. The storage and handling may be done in the nursery workroom or in another appropriate room in the hospital that is conveniently accessible at all hours. The preparation area shall have a work counter, a sink equipped for handwashing, and storage facilities.

7.4.G. Housekeeping/Environmental Services Room
A housekeeping/environmental services room shall be provided for the exclusive use of the nursery unit. It shall be directly accessible from the unit and shall contain a service sink or floor receptor and provide for storage of supplies and housekeeping equipment.

*7.5 Pediatric and Adolescent Unit

The unit shall meet the following standards:

7.5.A. Patient Rooms
Each patient room shall meet the following standards:

7.5.A1. Maximum room capacity shall be four patients.

7.5.A2. The space requirements for pediatric patient beds shall be the same as for adult beds due to the size variation and the need to change from cribs to beds, and vice-versa. See Section 7.2.A2 for requirements. Additional provisions for hygiene, toilets, sleeping, and personal belongings shall be included where the program indicates that parents will be allowed to remain with young children. (See Sections 7.3.D for pediatric critical care units and 7.4 for newborn nurseries.)

7.5.A3. Each patient room shall have a window in accordance with Section 7.28.A10.

7.5.B. Nursery
To minimize the possibility of cross infection, each nursery room serving pediatric patients shall contain no more than eight bassinets; each bassinet shall have a minimum clear floor area of 40 square feet (3.72 square meters). Each room shall contain a lavatory equipped for handwashing operable without hands, a nurses emergency calling system, and a glazed viewing window for observing infants from public areas and workrooms. (Limitation on number of patients in a nursery room does not apply to the pediatric critical care unit.)

7.5.C. Nursery Workrooms
Each nursery shall be served by a connecting workroom. It shall contain gowning facilities at the entrance for staff and housekeeping personnel; work space with a work counter; storage facilities; and a handwashing fixture. One workroom may serve more than one nursery.

7.5.D. Nursery Visiting and Feeding
Each pediatric nursery shall have an area for instruction and parent contact with the infant including breast and/or bottle feeding. This may be a section of the workroom with provisions for privacy and quiet.

7.5.E. Examination/Treatment Rooms
This room shall be provided for pediatric and adolescent patients. A separate area for infant examination and treatment may be provided within the pediatric nursery workroom. Examination/treatment rooms shall have a minimum floor area of 120 square feet (11.15 square meters). The room shall contain a handwashing fixture; storage facilities; and a desk, counter, or shelf space for writing.

7.5.F. Service Areas
The service areas in the pediatric and adolescent nursing units shall conform to Section 7.2.B and shall also meet the following standards:

7.5.F1. Multipurpose or individual room(s) shall be provided within or adjacent to areas serving pediatric and adolescent patrons for dining, education, and developmentally appropriate play and recreation, with access and equipment for patients with physical restrictions. If the functional program requires, an individual room shall be provided to allow for confidential parent/family comfort,

consultation, and teaching. Insulation, isolation, and structural provisions shall minimize the transmission of impact noise through the floor, walls, or ceiling of these multipurpose room(s).

7.5.F2. Space for preparation and storage of infant formula shall be provided within the unit or other convenient location. Provisions shall be made for continuation of special formula that may have been prescribed for the infant prior to admission or readmission.

7.5.F3. Patient toilet room(s) with handwashing facility(ies) in each room, in addition to those serving bed areas, shall be conveniently located to multipurpose room(s) and to each central bathing facility.

7.5.F4. Storage closets or cabinets for toys and educational and recreational equipment shall be provided.

7.5.F5. Storage space shall be provided to permit exchange of cribs and adult beds. Provisions shall also be made for storage of equipment and supplies (including cots or recliners, extra linen, etc.) for parents who stay with the patient overnight.

7.5.F6. At least one airborne infection isolation room shall be provided in each pediatric unit. The total number of infection isolation rooms shall be determined by an infection control risk assessment. Airborne infection isolation room(s) shall comply with the requirements of Section 7.2.C.

7.5.F7. Separate clean and soiled workrooms or holding rooms shall be provided as described in Sections 7.2.B11 and 12.

7.6 Psychiatric Nursing Unit

When part of a general hospital, these units shall be designed for the care of inpatients. Nonambulatory inpatients may be treated in a medical unit until their medical condition allows for transfer to the psychiatric nursing unit. See Section 7.2.E for psychiatric care in a medical unit. Provisions shall be made in the design for adapting the area for various types of psychiatric therapies.

The environment of the unit should be characterized by a feeling of openness with emphasis on natural light and exterior views. Various functions should be accessible from common areas while not compromising desirable levels of patient privacy. Interior finishes, lighting, and furnishings should suggest a residential rather than an institutional setting. These should, however, conform with applicable fire safety codes. Security and safety devices should not be presented in a manner to attract or challenge tampering by patients.

Windows or vents in psychiatric units shall be arranged and located so that they can be opened from the inside to permit venting of combustion products and to permit any occupant direct access to fresh air in emergencies. The operation of operable windows shall be restricted to inhibit possible escape or suicide. Where windows or vents require the use of tools or keys for operation, the tools or keys shall be located on the same floor in a prominent location accessible to staff. Windows in existing buildings designed with approved, engineered smoke control systems may be of fixed construction. Where glass fragments pose a hazard to certain patients, safety glazing and/or other appropriate security features shall be used.

Details of such facilities should be as described in the approved functional program. Each nursing unit shall provide the following:

7.6.A. Patient Rooms

The standard noted in Section 7.2.A shall apply to patient rooms in psychiatric nursing units except as follows:

7.6.A1. A nurses call system is not required, but if it is included, provisions shall be made for easy removal, or for covering call button outlets.

7.6.A2. Bedpan-flushing devices may be omitted from patient room toilets in psychiatric nursing units.

7.6.A3. Handwashing facilities are not required in patient rooms.

7.6.A4. Visual privacy in multibed rooms (e.g., cubicle curtains) is not required.

7.6.B. Service Areas

The standards noted in Section 7.2.B shall apply to service areas for psychiatric nursing units with the following modifications:

7.6.B1. A secured storage area shall be provided for patients' belongings that are determined to be potentially harmful (e.g., razors, nail files, cigarette lighters); this area will be controlled by staff.

7.6.B2. Medication station shall include provisions for security against unauthorized access.

7.6.B3. Food service within the unit may be one, or a combination, of the following:

a. A nourishment station.

b. A kitchenette designed for patient use with staff control of heating and cooking devices.

c. A kitchen service within the unit including a handwashing fixture, storage space, refrigerator, and facilities for meal preparation.

7.6.B4. Storage space for stretchers and wheelchairs may be outside the psychiatric unit, provided that provisions are made for convenient access as needed for disabled patients.

7.6.B5. In psychiatric nursing units, a bathtub or shower shall be provided for each six beds not otherwise served by bathing facilities within the patient rooms. Bathing facilities should be designed and located for patient convenience and privacy.

7.6.B6. A separate charting area shall be provided with provisions for acoustical privacy. A viewing window to permit observation of patient areas by the charting nurse or physician may be used if the arrangement is such that patient files cannot be read from outside the charting space.

7.6.B7. At least two separate social spaces, one appropriate for noisy activities and one for quiet activities, shall be provided. The combined area shall be at least 40 square feet (3.72 square meters) per patient with at least 120 square feet (11.15 square meters) for each of the two spaces. This space may be shared by dining activities.

7.6.B8. Space for group therapy shall be provided. This may be combined with the quiet space noted above when the unit accommodates not more than 12 patients, and when at least 225 square feet (20.92 square meters) of enclosed private space is available for group therapy activities.

7.6.B9. Patient laundry facilities with an automatic washer and dryer shall be provided.

The following elements shall also be provided, but may be either within the psychiatric unit or immediately accessible to it unless otherwise dictated by the program:

7.6.B10. Room(s) for examination and treatment with a minimum area of 120 square feet (11.15 square meters). Examination and treatment room(s) for medical-surgical patients may be shared by the psychiatric unit patients. (These may be on a different floor if conveniently accessible.)

7.6.B11. Separate consultation room(s) with minimum floor space of 100 square feet (9.29 square meters) each, provided at a room-to-bed ratio of one consultation room for each 12 psychiatric beds. The room(s) shall be designed for acoustical and visual privacy and constructed to achieve a noise reduction of at least 45 decibels.

7.6.B12. Psychiatric units each containing 15 square feet (1.39 square meters) of separate space per patient for occupational therapy, with a minimum total area of at least 200 square feet (18.58 square meters), whichever is greater. Space shall include provision for handwashing, work counter(s), storage, and displays. Occupational therapy areas may serve more than one nursing unit. When psychiatric nursing unit(s) contain less than 12 beds, the occupational therapy functions may be performed within the noisy activities area, if at least an additional 10 square feet (0.93 square meter) per patient served is included.

7.6.B13. A conference and treatment planning room for use by the psychiatric unit.

7.6.C. Airborne Infection Isolation Room(s)

At least one airborne infection isolation room shall be provided in the psychiatric unit. The room designated for isolation in the psychiatric unit may be the seclusion room with appropriate safety precautions. The total number of infection isolation rooms shall be determined by an infection control risk assessment. Airborne infection isolation room(s) shall comply with the requirements of Section 7.2.C.

7.6.D. Seclusion Treatment Room

There shall be at least one seclusion room for up to 24 beds or a major fraction thereof. The seclusion treatment room is intended for short-term occupancy by a violent or suicidal patient. Within the psychiatric nursing unit, this space provides for patients requiring security and protection. The room(s) shall be located for direct nursing staff supervision. Each room shall be for only one patient. It shall have an area of at least 60 square feet (5.57 square meters) and shall be constructed to prevent patient hiding, escape, injury, or suicide. Where restraint beds are required by the functional program, 80 square feet (7.43 square meters) shall be required. If a facility has more than one psychiatric nursing unit, the number of seclusion rooms shall be a function of the total number of psychiatric beds in the facility. Seclusion rooms may be grouped together. Special fixtures and hardware for electrical circuits shall be used. Minimum ceiling height shall be 9 feet (2.74 meters). Doors shall be 3 feet 8 inches (1.12 meters) wide, and shall permit staff observation of the patient while also maintaining provisions for patient privacy. Seclusion treatment rooms shall be accessed by an anteroom or vestibule which also provides direct access to a toilet room. The toilet room and anteroom shall be large enough to safely manage the patient.

Where the interior of the seclusion treatment room is padded with combustible materials, these materials shall be of a type acceptable to the local authority having jurisdiction. The room area, including floor, walls, ceilings, and all openings shall be protected with not less than one-hour-rated construction.

7.7 Surgical Suites

Note: The number of operating rooms and recovery beds and the sizes of the service areas shall be based on the expected surgical workload. In the program, the size, location, and configuration of the surgical suite and support service departments shall reflect the projected volume of outpatients. This may be achieved by designing either an outpatient surgery facility or a combined inpatient-outpatient surgical suite. The surgical suite shall be located and arranged to prevent nonrelated traffic through the suite.

When bronchoscopy is performed on persons who are known or suspected of having pulmonary tuberculosis, the procedure room shall meet the airborne infection isolation room ventilation requirements.

When invasive procedures are performed on persons who are known or suspected of having airborne infectious disease, these procedures should not be performed in the operating suite. They shall be performed in a room meeting airborne infection isolation ventilation requirements or in a space using local exhaust ventilation. If the procedure must be performed in the operating suite, see the CDC's "Guidelines for Preventing the Transmission of Mycobacterium Tuberculosis in Health Care Facilities."

Additions to, and adaptations of, the following elements shall be made for the special-procedure operating rooms found in larger facilities.

The following shall be provided:

7.7.A. Surgery

7.7.A1. General operating room(s). In new construction, each room shall have a minimum clear area of 400 square feet (37.16 square meters) exclusive of fixed or wall-mounted cabinets and built-in shelves, with a minimum of 20 feet (6.10 meters) clear dimension between fixed cabinets and built-in shelves; and a system for emergency communication with the surgical suite control station. X-ray film illuminators for handling at least four films simultaneously shall also be provided. Where renovation work is undertaken, every effort shall be made to meet the above minimum standards. If it is not possible to meet the above square-foot standards, the authorities having jurisdiction may grant approval to deviate from this requirement. In such cases, each room shall have a minimum clear area of 360 square feet (33.45 square meters), exclusive of fixed or wall-mounted cabinets and built-in shelves, with a minimum of 18 feet (5.49 meters) clear dimension between fixed cabinets and built-in shelves. (For renovation projects, see Section 7.7.A6.)

7.7.A2. Room(s) for cardiovascular, orthopedic, neurological, and other special procedures that require additional personnel and/or large equipment. When included, this room shall have, in addition to the above, a minimum clear area of 600 square feet (55.74 square meters), with a minimum of 20 feet (6.10 meters) clear dimension exclusive of fixed or wall-mounted cabinets and built-in shelves. When open-heart surgery is performed, an additional room in the restricted area of the surgical suite, preferably adjoining this operating room, shall be designated as a pump room where extra corporeal pump(s), supplies and accessories are stored and serviced. When complex orthopedic and neurosurgical surgery is performed, additional rooms shall be in the restricted area of the surgical suite, preferably adjoining the specialty operating rooms, which shall be designated as equipment storage rooms for the large equipment used to support these procedures. Appropriate plumbing and electrical connections shall be provided in the cardiovascular, orthopedic, neurosurgical, pump, and storage rooms. Where renovation work is undertaken, every effort shall be made to meet the above minimum standards. If it is not possible to meet the above square-foot standards, the authorities having jurisdiction may grant approval to deviate from this requirement. In such cases, orthopedic surgical rooms may have a minimum clear area of 360 square feet (33.48 square meters) and a minimum dimension of 18 feet (5.49 meters). Rooms for cardiovascular, neurological, and other special procedures may have a minimum clear area of 400 square feet (37.16 square meters).

7.7.A3. A room for orthopedic surgery. When included, this room shall, in addition to the above, have enclosed storage space for splints and traction equipment. Storage may be outside the operating room but must be conveniently located. If a sink is used for the disposal of plaster of paris, a plaster trap shall be provided.

7.7.A4. Room(s) for surgical cystoscopic and other endo-urologic procedures. This room shall have a minimum clear area of 350 square feet (32.52 square meters) exclusive of fixed or wall-mounted cabinets and built-in shelves with a minimum of 15 feet (4.57 meters) clear dimension between fixed cabinets and built-in shelves. X-ray viewing capability to accommodate at least four films simultaneously will be provided. In renovation projects, rooms for surgical cystoscopy may have a minimum clear area of 250 square feet (23.28 square meters).

7.7.A5. Endoscopy suite requirements. (See Section 9.9.)

7.7.A6. The functional program may require additional clear space, plumbing, and mechanical facilities to accommodate special functions in one or more of these rooms. When existing functioning operating rooms are modified, and it is impractical to increase the square foot area because of walls or structural members, the operating room may continue in use when requested by the hospital.

7.7.B1. Preoperative patient holding area(s). In facilities with two or more operating rooms, areas shall be provided to accommodate stretcher patients as well as sitting space for ambulatory patients not requiring stretchers. These areas shall be under the visual control of the nursing staff.

*7.7.B2. Post-Anesthetic Care Units (PACUs)
Each PACU shall contain a medication station; handwashing facilities; nurse station with charting facilities; clinical sink; provisions for bedpan cleaning; and storage space for stretchers, supplies, and equipment. Additionally, the design shall provide a minimum of 80 square feet (7.43 square meters) for each patient bed with a space for additional equipment described in the functional program, and for clearance of at least 4 feet (1.22 meters) between patient beds and between patient bedsides and adjacent walls. Provisions shall be made for the isolation of infectious patients. Provisions for patient privacy such as cubicle curtains shall be made. In new construction, at least one door to the recovery room shall access directly from the surgical suite without crossing public hospital corridors.

An airborne infection isolation room is not required in a PACU. Provisions for the recovery of a potentially infectious patient with an airborne infection shall be determined by the infection control risk assessment.

A staff toilet shall be located within the working area to maintain staff availability to patients.

Handwashing facilities with hands-free operable controls shall be available with at least one for every four beds uniformly distributed to provide equal access from each patient bed.

7.7.C. Service Areas
Services, except for the enclosed soiled workroom mentioned in item 7.7.C6 and the housekeeping room in item 7.7.C19, may be shared with the obstetrical facilities if the functional program reflects this concept. Service areas, when shared with delivery rooms, shall be designed to avoid the passing of patients or staff between the operating room and the delivery room areas. The following services shall be provided:

7.7.C1. A control station located to permit visual observation of all traffic into the suite.

7.7.C2. A supervisor's office or station.

7.7.C3. A sterilizing facility(ies) with high-speed sterilizer(s) or other sterilizing equipment for immediate or emergency use must be grouped to several operating rooms for convenient, efficient use. A work space and handwashing facility may be included. Other facilities for processing and sterilizing reusable instruments, etc., may be located in another hospital department such as central services.

7.7.C4. Medication station. Provision shall be made for storage and distribution of drugs and routine medications. This may be done from a medicine preparation room or unit, from a self-contained medicine dispensing unit, or by another system. If used, a medicine preparation room or unit shall be under visual control of nursing staff. It shall contain a work counter, sink, refrigerator, and double-locked storage for controlled substances. Convenient access to handwashing facilities shall be provided. (Standard cup-sinks provided in many self-contained units are not adequate for handwashing.)

7.7.C5. Scrub facilities. Two scrub positions shall be provided near the entrance to each operating room. Two scrub positions may serve two operating rooms if both are located adjacent to the entrance of each operating room. Scrub facilities should be arranged to minimize incidental splatter on nearby personnel, medical equipment, or supply carts. In new construction, view windows at scrub stations permitting observation of room interiors should be provided. The scrub sinks should be recessed into an alcove out of the main traffic areas. The alcove shall be located off the semirestricted or restricted areas of the surgical suite. Scrub sinks shall be located outside the sterile core.

7.7.C6. An enclosed soiled workroom (or soiled holding room that is part of a system for the collection and disposal of soiled material) for the exclusive use of the surgical suite shall be provided. It shall be located in the restricted area. The soiled workroom shall contain a flushing-rim clinical sink or equivalent flushing-rim fixture, a handwashing fixture, a work counter, and space for waste receptacles and soiled linen receptacles. Rooms used only for temporary holding of soiled material may omit the flushing-rim clinical sink and work counters. However, if the flushing-rim clinical sink is omitted, other provisions for disposal of liquid waste shall be provided. The room shall not have direct connection with operating rooms or other sterile activity rooms. Soiled and clean workrooms or holding rooms shall be separated.

7.7.C7. Clean workroom or clean supply room.

a. A clean workroom is required when clean materials are assembled within the surgical suite prior to use or following the decontamination cycle. It shall contain a work counter, a handwashing fixture, storage facilities for clean supplies, and a space to package reusable items. The storage for sterile supplies must be separated from this space. If the room is used only for storage and holding as part of a system for distribution of clean and sterile supply materials, the work counter and handwashing fixture may be omitted. Soiled and clean workrooms or holding rooms shall be separated.

b. Storage space for sterile and clean supplies should be adequate for the functional plan. The space should be moisture and temperature controlled and free from cross traffic.

c. An operating room suite design with a sterile core must provide for no cross traffic of staff and supplies from the decontaminated/soiled areas to the sterile/clean areas. The use of facilities outside the operating room for soiled/decontaminated processing and clean assembly and sterile processing will be designed to move the flow of goods and personnel from dirty to clean/sterile without compromising universal precautions or aseptic techniques in both departments.

7.7.C8. Medical gas storage facilities. Main storage of medical gases may be outside or inside the facility in accordance with NFPA 99. Provision shall be made for additional separate storage of reserve gas cylinders necessary to complete at least one day's procedures.

7.7.C9. The anesthesia workroom for cleaning, testing, and storing anesthesia equipment shall contain work counter(s) and sink(s) and racks for cylinders. Provisions shall be made for separate storage of clean and soiled items. In new construction, depending on the functional and space programs, the anesthesia workroom should provide space for anesthesia case carts and other anesthesia equipment.

7.7.C10. Equipment storage room(s) for equipment and supplies used in surgical suite.

7.7.C11. Staff clothing change areas. Appropriate areas shall be provided for male and female personnel (orderlies, technicians, nurses, and doctors) working within the surgical suite. The areas shall contain lockers, showers, toilets, lavatories equipped for handwashing, and space for donning surgical attire. These areas shall be arranged to encourage a one-way traffic pattern so that personnel entering from outside the surgical suite can change and move directly into the surgical suite.

7.7.C12. Staff lounge and toilet facilities. Separate or combined lounges for male and female staff shall be provided. Lounge(s) shall be designed to minimize the need to leave the suite and to provide convenient access to the recovery room.

7.7.C13. Dictation and report preparation area. This may be accessible from the lounge area.

7.7.C14. Outpatient recovery. If the functional program includes outpatient surgery, provisions shall be made for separating outpatients into two categories, (Phase I) patients receiving general anesthesia and (Phase II) patients not subjected to general anesthesia. This requirement should be satisfied by separate rooms. Phase II shall provide privacy for each patient. A patient toilet room directly accessible from outpatient recovery shall be provided. Smaller facilities with no more than two surgical procedure rooms may use the same space for (Phase II) recovery of patient not subjected to general anesthesia as that used for preoperative preparation.

7.7.C15. Change areas for outpatients and same-day admissions. If the functional program defines outpatient surgery as part of the surgical suite, a separate area shall be provided where outpatients may change from street clothing into hospital gowns and be prepared for surgery. This would include a waiting room, locker(s), toilet(s), and clothing change or gowning area. Changing may also be accommodated in a private holding room or cubicle.

7.7.C16. Provisions shall be made for patient examination, interviews, preparation, testing, and obtaining vital signs of patients for outpatient surgery.

7.7.C18. Storage areas for portable X-ray equipment, stretchers, fracture tables, warming devices, auxiliary lamps, etc. These areas shall be out of corridors and traffic.

7.7.C19. Housekeeping facilities. Housekeeping facilities shall be provided for the exclusive use of the surgical suite. It shall be directly accessible from the suite and shall contain a service sink or floor receptor and provisions for storage of supplies and housekeeping equipment.

7.7.C20. Area for preparation and examination of frozen sections. This may be part of the general laboratory if immediate results are obtainable without unnecessary delay in the completion of surgery.

7.7.C21. Ice machine. An ice machine shall be provided to provide ice for treatments and patient use. Ice intended for human consumption shall be from self-dispensing ice makers.

7.7.C22. Provisions for refrigerated blood bank storage.

7.7.C23. Where applicable, appropriate provisions for refrigeration facilities for harvested organs.

7.7.C24. Provisions for pathological specimens storage prior to transfer to pathology section.

7.7.C25. See Section 9.5 of this document concerning the separate outpatient surgical unit.

*7.8 Obstetrical Facilities (See Appendix A)

7.8.A. Obstetrical Suite

7.8.A1. General
The obstetrical unit shall be located and designed to prohibit non-related traffic through the unit. When delivery and operating rooms are in the same suite, access and service arrangements shall be such that neither staff nor patients need to travel through one area to reach the other. Except as permitted otherwise herein, existing facilities being renovated shall, as far as practicable, provide all the required support services.

7.8.A2. Postpartum Unit
a. Postpartum bedroom

(1) A postpartum bedroom shall have a minimum of 100 square feet (9.29 square meters) of clear floor area per bed in multi-bedded rooms and 120 square feet (11.15 square meters) of clear floor area in single-bed rooms. These areas shall be exclusive of toilet rooms, closets, alcoves, or vestibules. Where renovation work is undertaken, every effort shall be made to meet the above minimum standards. If it is not possible to meet the above square-foot standards, the authorities having jurisdiction

may grant approval to deviate from this requirement. In such cases, existing postpartum patient rooms shall have no less than 80 square feet (7.43 square meters) of clear floor area per bed in multiple-bed rooms and 100 square feet (9.29 square meters) in single-bed rooms.

(2) In multi-bedded rooms there shall be a minimum clear distance of 4 feet (1.22 meters) between the foot of the bed and the opposite wall, 3 feet (0.91 meter) between the side of the bed and the nearest wall, and 4 feet (1.22 meters) between beds.

(3) The maximum number of beds per room shall be two.

(4) Each patient bedroom shall have a window or windows that can be opened from the inside. When the windows require the use of tools or keys, they shall be kept on the unit and readily accessible to staff.

(5) Handwashing facilities shall be provided in each patient bedroom. In multi-bedded rooms the handwashing sink shall be located outside of the patients' cubical curtains so that it is accessible to staff.

(6) Each patient shall have access to a toilet room or bathroom with handwashing facilities without entering a general corridor. One such room shall serve no more than two beds and no more than two patient rooms.

b. The following support services for this unit shall be provided.

(1) A nurse station.

(2) A nurse office.

(3) Charting facilities.

(4) Toilet room for staff.

(5) Staff lounge.

(6) Lockable closets or cabinets for personal articles of staff.

(7) Consultation/conference room(s).

(8) Patients' lounge. The patients' lounge may be omitted if all rooms are single-bed rooms.

(9) Clean workroom or clean supply room. A clean workroom is required if clean materials are assembled within the obstetrical suite prior to use. It shall contain a work counter, a handwashing fixture, and storage facilities for clean and sterile supplies. If the room is used only for storage and holding as part of a system for distribution of clean and sterile supply materials, the work counter and handwashing fixtures may be omitted. Soiled and clean workrooms or holding rooms shall be separated and have no direct connection.

(10) Soiled workroom or soiled holding room for the exclusive use of the obstetrical suite. This room shall be separate from the clean workroom. The soiled workroom

shall contain a clinical sink (or equivalent flushing-rim fixture) and a handwashing fixture. The above fixtures shall have a hot and cold mixing faucet. The room shall have a work counter and space for separate covered containers for soiled linen and waste. Rooms used only for temporary holding of soiled material may omit the clinical sink and work counter. If the flushing-rim clinical sink is omitted, facilities for cleaning bedpans shall be provided elsewhere.

(11) Medication station. Provision shall be made for storage and distribution of drugs and routine medications. This may be done from a medicine preparation room or unit, from a self-contained medicine dispensing unit, or by another system. If used, a medicine preparation room or unit shall be under visual control of nursing staff. It shall contain a work counter, sink, refrigerator, and double-locked storage for controlled substances. Convenient access to handwashing facilities shall be provided. (Standard cup-sinks provided in many self-contained units are not adequate for handwashing.)

(12) Clean linen storage may be part of a clean workroom or a separate closet. When a closed cart system is used, the cart may be stored in a alcove out of the path of normal traffic.

(13) Nourishment station shall contain sink, work counter, ice dispenser, refrigerator, cabinets, and equipment for serving hot or cold food. Space shall be included for temporary holding of unused or soiled dietary trays.

(14) Equipment storage room.

(15) Storage space for stretchers and wheelchairs. Storage space for stretchers and wheelchairs shall be provided in a strategic location, out of corridors and away from normal traffic.

(16) When bathing facilities are not provided in patient rooms, there shall be at least one shower and/or bathtub for each 6 beds or fraction thereof.

(17) Housekeeping room. A housekeeping room shall be provided for the exclusive use of the obstetrical suite. It shall be directly accessible from the suite and shall contain a service sink or floor receptor and provisions for storage of supplies and housekeeping equipment.

(18) Examination/treatment room and/or multipurpose diagnostic testing room shall have a minimum clear floor area of 120 square feet (11.15 square meters). When utilized as a multipatient diagnostic testing room, a minimum clear floor area of 80 square feet (7.43 square meters) per patient shall be provided. An adjoining toilet room shall be provided for patient use.

(19) Emergency equipment storage shall be located in close proximity to the nurse station.

c. Airborne infection isolation room(s). An airborne infection isolation room is not required for the obstetrical unit. Provisions for the care of the perinatal patient with an airborne infection shall be determined by the infection control risk assessment.

7.8.A3. Caesarean/Delivery Suite
a. Caesarean/delivery room(s) shall have a minimum clear floor area of 360 square feet (33.45 square meters) with a minimum dimension of 16 feet (4.88 meters) exclusive of built-in shelves or cabinets. There shall be a minimum of one such room in every obstetrical unit.

b. Delivery room(s) shall have a minimum clear area of 300 square feet (27.87 square meters) exclusive of fixed cabinets and built-in shelves. An emergency communication system shall be connected with the obstetrical suite control station.

c. Infant resuscitation shall be provided within the caesarean/delivery room(s) and delivery rooms with a minimum clear floor area of 40 square feet (3.72 square meters) in addition to the required area of each room or may be provided in a separate but immediately accessible room with a clear floor area of 150 square feet (13.94 square meters). Six single or three duplex electrical outlets shall be provided for the infant in addition to the facilities required for the mother.

d. Labor room(s) (LDR rooms may be substituted). In renovation projects, existing labor rooms may have a minimum clear area of 100 square feet (9.29 square meters) per bed.

Where LDRs or LDRPs are not provided, a minimum of two labor beds shall be provided for each caesarean/delivery room. In facilities that have only one caesarean/delivery room, two labor rooms shall be provided. Each room shall be designed for either one or two beds with a minimum clear area of 120 square feet (11.15 square meters) per bed. Each labor room shall contain a handwashing fixture and have access to a toilet room. One toilet room may serve two labor rooms. Labor rooms shall have controlled access with doors that are arranged for observation from a nursing station. At least one shower (which may be separate from the labor room if under staff control) for use of patients in labor shall be provided. Windows in labor rooms, if provided, shall be located, draped, or otherwise arranged to preserve patient privacy from casual observation from outside the labor room.

e. Recovery room(s) (LDR rooms may be substituted). Each recovery room shall contain at least two beds and have a nurse station with charting facilities located to permit visual control of all beds. Each room shall include facilities for handwashing and dispensing medicine. A clinical sink with bedpan flushing device shall be available, as shall storage for supplies and equipment. There should be enough space for baby and crib and a chair for the support person. There should be the ability to maintain visual privacy of the new family.

f. Service areas

(1) Individual rooms shall be provided as indicated in the following standards; otherwise, alcoves or other open spaces that do not interfere with traffic may be used.

(2) The following services shall be provided:

(a) A control/nurse station located to restrict unauthorized traffic into the suite.

(b) Soiled workroom or soiled holding room. This room shall be separate from the clean workroom. The soiled workroom shall contain a clinical sink (or equivalent flushing-rim fixture). The room shall contain a handwashing fixture. The above fixtures shall have a hot and cold mixing faucet. The room shall have a work counter and space for separate covered containers for soiled linen and waste. Rooms used only for temporary holding of soiled material may omit the clinical sink and work counter. If the flushing-rim clinical sink is eliminated, facilities for cleaning bedpans shall be provided elsewhere.

(c) Fluid waste disposal.

(3) The following services may be shared with the surgical facilities if the functional program reflects this concern. When shared, areas shall be arranged to avoid direct traffic between the delivery and operating rooms

(a) A supervisor's office or station.

(b) A waiting room, with toilets, telephones, and drinking fountains conveniently located. The toilet room shall contain handwashing facilities.

(c) Sterilizing facilities with high-speed sterilizers convenient to all caesarean/delivery rooms. Sterilization facilities should be separate from the delivery area and adjacent to clean assembly. High-speed autoclaves should only be used in an emergency situation (i.e., a dropped instrument and no sterile replacement readily available). Sterilization facilities would not be necessary if the flow of materials were handled properly from a central service department based on the usage of the delivery room (DR).

(d) A drug distribution station with handwashing facilities and provisions for controlled storage, preparation, and distribution of medication.

(e) Scrub facilities for caesarean/delivery rooms. Two scrub positions shall be provided adjacent to entrance to each caesarean/delivery room. Scrub facilities should be arranged to minimize any splatter on nearby personnel or supply carts. In new construction, provide view windows at scrub stations to permit the observation of room interiors.

(f) Clean workroom or clean supply room. A clean workroom shall be provided if clean materials are assembled within the obstetrical suite prior to use. If a clean workroom is provided it shall contain a work counter, sink equipped for handwashing, and space for storage of supplies. A clean supply room may be provided when the functional program defines a system for the storage and distribution of clean and sterile supplies. See (h) below for sterile storage.

(g) Medical gas storage facilities. See Section 7.7.C8.

(h) A clean sterile storage area readily available to the DR: size to be determined on level of usage, functions provided, and supplies from the hospital central distribution area.

(i) An anesthesia workroom for cleaning, testing, and storing anesthesia equipment. It shall contain a work counter, sink, and provisions for separation of clean and soiled items.

(j) Equipment storage room(s) for equipment and supplies used in the obstetrical suite.

(k) Staff clothing change areas. The clothing change area shall be designed to minimize physical contact between clean and contaminated personnel. The area shall contain lockers, showers, toilets, handwashing facilities, and space for donning and disposing scrub suits and booties.

(l) Male and female support persons change area (designed as described above.)

(m) Lounge and toilet facilities for obstetrical staff convenient to delivery, labor, and recovery areas. The toilet room shall contain handwashing facilities.

(n) An on-call room(s) for physician and/or staff may be located elsewhere in the facility.

(o) Housekeeping room with a floor receptacle or service sink and storage space for housekeeping supplies and equipment.

(p) An area for storing stretchers out of the path of normal traffic.

7.8.A4. LDR and LDRP Facilities
When provided by the functional program, delivery procedures in accordance with birthing concepts may be performed in the LDR or LDRP rooms. LDR room(s) may be located in a separate LDR suite or as part of the Caesarean/Delivery suite. The postpartum unit may contain LDRP rooms. These rooms shall have a minimum of 250 square feet (23.28 square meters) of clear floor area with a minimum dimension of 13 feet (3.96 meters), exclusive of toilet room, closet, alcove, or vestibules. There should be enough space for crib and reclining chair for support person. An area within the room but distinct from the mother's area shall be provided for infant stabilization and resuscitation. See Table 5 for

medical gas outlets. These outlets should be located in the room so that they are accessible to the mother's delivery area and infant resuscitation area. When renovation work is undertaken, every effort shall be made to meet the above minimum standards. If it is not possible to meet the above square-foot standards, the authorities having jurisdiction may grant approval to deviate from this requirement. In such cases, existing LDR or LDRP rooms may have a minimum clear area of 200 square feet (18.58 square meters).

Each LDR or LDRP room shall be for single occupancy and have direct access to a private toilet with shower or tub. Each room shall be equipped with handwashing facilities (handwashing facilities with hands-free operation are acceptable for scrubbing). Examination lights may be portable, but must be immediately accessible.

Finishes shall be selected to facilitate cleaning and with resistance to strong detergents. Windows or doors within a normal sightline that would permit observation into the room shall be arranged or draped as necessary for patient privacy.

7.9 Emergency Service

(See Section 9.6 for the separate outpatient emergency unit.)

*7.9.A. Definition
Levels of emergency care range from initial emergency management to definitive emergency care. For classification of emergency departments/services/trauma centers, see Appendix A.

7.9.A1. Initial emergency management is care provided to stabilize a victim's condition and to minimize potential for further injury during transport to an appropriate service. Patients may be brought to the "nearest hospital," which may or may not have all required services for definitive emergency management. It is important that the hospital, in those cases, be able to assess and stabilize emergent illnesses and injuries and arrange for appropriate transfer.

7.9.A2. Emergency care may range from the suturing of lacerations to full-scale emergency medical procedures. Facilities that include personnel and equipment for definitive emergency care should provide for 24-hour service and complete emergency care leading to discharge to the patient's home or direct admission to the appropriate hospital.

7.9.B. General
The extent and type of emergency service to be provided will depend upon community needs and the availability of other services within the area. While initial emergency management must be available at every hospital, full-scale definitive emergency services may be impractical and/or an unnecessary duplication. All services need adequate equipment and 24-hour staffing to ensure no delay in essential treatment. The following standards are intended only as minimums. Additional facilities, as needed, shall be as required to satisfy the program.

Provisions for facilities to provide nonemergency treatment of outpatients are covered separately in Section 9.3.

7.9.C. Initial Emergency Management
At a minimum, each hospital shall have provisions for emergency treatment for staff, employees, and visitors, as well as for persons who may be unaware of or unable to immediately reach services in other facilities. This is not only for patients with minor illnesses or injuries that may require minimal care but also for persons with severe illness and injuries who must receive immediate emergency care and assistance prior to transport to other facilities.

Provisions for initial emergency management shall include:

7.9.C1. A well-marked, illuminated, and covered entrance, at grade level.

Reception, triage, and control station shall be located to permit staff observation and control of access to treatment area, pedestrian and ambulance entrances, and public waiting area.

7.9.C2. A treatment room with not less than 120 square feet (11.15 square meters) of clear area, exclusive of toilets, waiting area, and storage. Each treatment room shall contain an examination light, work counter, handwashing facilities, medical equipment, cabinets, medication storage, adequate electrical outlets above floor level, and counter space for writing. The treatment room may have additional space and provisions for several patients with cubicle curtains for privacy. Multiple-bed treatment rooms shall provide a minimum of 80 square feet (7.43 square meters) per patient cubicle.

7.9.C3. Storage out of traffic and under staff control for general medical/surgical emergency supplies, medications, and equipment such as ventilator, defibrillator, splints, etc.

7.9.C4. Provisions for reception, control, and public waiting, including a public toilet with handwashing facility(ies), and telephone.

7.9.C5. A patient toilet room with handwashing facility(ies) convenient to the treatment room(s).

7.9.C6. Communication hookup to the Poison Control Center and regional EMS system.

*7.9.C7. Airborne infection control.

7.9.D. Definitive Emergency Care

When 24-hour emergency service is to be provided, the type, size, and number of the services shall be as defined in the functional program. As a minimum, the following shall be provided:

7.9.D1. Grade-level well-marked, illuminated, and covered entrance with direct access from public roads for ambulance and vehicle traffic. Entrance and driveway shall be clearly marked. If a raised platform is used for ambulance discharge, provide a ramp for pedestrian and wheelchair access.

7.9.D2. Paved emergency access to permit discharge of patients from automobiles and ambulances, and temporary parking convenient to the entrance.

7.9.D3. Reception, triage (see Table 5 in Section 7.31), and control station shall be located to permit staff observation and control of access to treatment area, pedestrian and ambulance entrances, and public waiting area.

The triage area requires special consideration. As the point of entry and assessment for patients with undiagnosed and untreated airborne infections, the triage area shall be designed and ventilated to reduce exposure of staff, patients and families to airborne infectious diseases. If determined by the infection control risk assessment, one or more separate, enclosed spaces designed and ventilated as airborne infection isolation rooms shall be required.

7.9.D4. Wheelchair and stretcher storage shall be provided for arriving patients. This shall be out of traffic with convenient access from emergency entrances.

7.9.D5. Public waiting area with toilet facilities, drinking fountains, and telephones shall be provided. If so determined by the hospital infection control risk assessment, the emergency department waiting area shall require special measures to reduce the risk of airborne infection transmission. These measures may include enhanced general ventilation and air disinfection similar to inpatient requirements for airborne infection isolation rooms. See the CDC's "Guidelines for Preventing the Transmission of Mycobacterium Tuberculosis in Health Care Facilities."

7.9.D6. Communication center shall be convenient to nursing station and have radio, telephone, and intercommunication systems. (See Section 7.29.F.)

7.9.D7. Examination and treatment room(s). Examination rooms shall have a minimum floor area of 120 square feet (11.15 square meters). The room shall contain work counter(s); cabinets; handwashing facilities; supply storage facilities; examination lights; a desk, counter, or shelf space for writing; and a vision panel adjacent to and/or in the door. When treatment cubicles are in open multiple-bed areas, each cubicle shall have a minimum of 80 square feet (7.43 square meters) of clear floor space and shall be separated from adjoining cubicles by curtains. Handwashing facilities shall be provided for each four treatment cubicles or major fraction thereof in multiple-bed areas. For oxygen and vacuum, see Table 5 in Section 7.31. Treatment/examination rooms used for pelvic exams should allow for the foot of the examination table to face away from the door.

*7.9.D8. Trauma/cardiac rooms for emergency procedures, including emergency surgery, shall have at least 250 square feet (23.28 square meters) of clear floor space. Each room shall have cabinets and emergency supply shelves, X-ray film illuminators, examination lights, and counter space for writing. Additional space with cubicle curtains for privacy may be provided to accommodate more than one patient at a time in the trauma room. Provisions shall be made for monitoring the patient. There shall be storage provided for immediate access to attire used for universal precautions. Doorways leading from the ambulance entrance to the cardiac trauma room shall be a minimum of 5 feet (1.52 meters) wide to simultaneously accommodate stretchers, equipment, and personnel. In renovation projects, every effort shall be made to have existing cardiac/trauma rooms meet the above minimum standards. If it is not possible to meet the above square-foot standards, the authorities having jurisdiction may grant approval to deviate from this requirement. In such cases, these rooms shall be no less than a clear area of 240 square feet (22.32 square meters), and doorways leading from the ambulance entrance to the room may be 4 feet (1.22 meters) wide.

7.9.D9. Provisions for orthopedic and cast work. These may be in separate room(s) or in the trauma room. They shall include storage for splints and other orthopedic supplies, traction hooks, X-ray film illuminators, and examination lights. If a sink is used for the disposal of plaster of paris, a plaster trap shall be provided. The clear floor space for this area shall depend on the functional program and the procedures and equipment accommodated here.

7.9.D10. Scrub stations located in or adjacent and convenient to each trauma and/or orthopedic room.

7.9.D11. Convenient access to radiology and laboratory services.

7.9.D12. Poison Control Center and EMS Communications Center may be a part of the staff work and charting area.

7.9.D13. Provisions for disposal of solid and liquid waste. This may be a clinical sink with bedpan flushing device within the soiled workroom.

7.9.D14. Emergency equipment storage. Sufficient space shall be provided for emergency equipment that is under direct control of the nursing staff, such as a CPR cart, pumps, ventilators, patient monitoring equipment, and portable X-ray unit. This space shall be located in an area appropriate to the functional program easily accessible to staff but out of normal traffic patterns.

7.9.D15. A toilet room for patients. When there are more than eight treatment areas, a minimum of two toilet facilities, with handwashing facility(ies) in each toilet room, will be required.

7.9.D16. Storage rooms for clean, soiled, or used supplies.

*a. Soiled workroom or soiled holding room for the exclusive use of the emergency service. This room shall be separate from the clean workroom. The soiled workroom shall contain a clinical sink (or equivalent flushing-rim fixture). The room shall contain a lavatory (or handwashing fixture). The above fixtures shall both have a hot and cold mixing faucet. The room shall have a work counter and space for separate covered containers for soiled linen and waste. Rooms used only for temporary holding of soiled material may omit the clinical sink and work counter. If the flushing-rim clinical sink is eliminated, facilities for cleaning bedpans shall be provided elsewhere.

b. Clean workroom or clean supply room. If the room is used for preparing patient care items, it shall contain a work counter, a handwashing sink, and storage facilities for clean and sterile supplies. If the room is used only for storage and holding as part of a system for distribution of clean and sterile supply materials, the work counter and handwashing facilities may be omitted. If the area serves children, additional storage shall be provided to accommodate supplies and equipment in the range of sizes required for pediatrics. Soiled and clean workrooms or holding rooms shall be separated and have no direct connection.

7.9.D17. Administrative center or nurses station for staff work and charting. These areas shall have space for counters, cabinets, and medication storage, and shall have convenient access to handwashing facilities. They may be combined with or include centers for reception and communication or poison control. These nursing stations may also be decentralized near clusters of treatment rooms. Visual observation of all traffic into the unit and of all patients should be provided from the nursing station, where feasible.

7.9.D18. Securable closets or cabinet compartments for the personal effects of emergency service personnel, located in or near the nurse station. At a minimum, these shall be large enough for purses and billfolds. Coats may be stored in closets or cabinets in the unit or in a central staff locker area.

7.9.D19. Staff lounge. Convenient and private access to staff toilets, lounge, and lockers shall be provided.

7.9.D20. Housekeeping room. A housekeeping room shall be provided for the exclusive use of the emergency service. It shall be directly accessible from the unit and shall contain a service sink or floor receptor and provisions for storage of supplies and housekeeping equipment.

*7.9.D21. Security Station
The non-selective 24-hour accessibility of the emergency department dictates that a security system reflecting local community needs be provided.

7.9.D22. Airborne Infection Isolation Room
At least one airborne infection isolation room shall be provided as described in Section 7.2.C. The need for additional airborne infection isolation rooms or for protective environment rooms as described in Section 7.2.D shall be determined by the infection control risk assessment.

*7.9.D23. Bereavement Room.

7.9.D24. Secured Holding Room
At least one holding/seclusion room of 120 square feet (11.15 square meters) shall be provided. This room shall allow for security, patient and staff safety, patient observation, and soundproofing.

*7.9.E. Other Space Considerations

7.10 Imaging Suite

7.10.A. General

7.10.A1. Equipment and space shall be as necessary to accommodate the functional program. The imaging department provides diagnostic procedures. It includes fluoroscopy, radiography, mammography, tomography, computerized tomography scanning, ultrasound, magnetic resonance, angiography, and other similar techniques. Layouts should be developed in compliance with manufacturer's recommendations, because area requirements may vary from machine to machine. Since technology changes frequently and from manufacturer to manufacturer, rooms can be sized larger to allow upgrading of equipment over a period of time.

7.10.A2. Most imaging requires radiation protection. A certified physicist or other qualified expert representing the owner or appropriate state agency shall specify the type, location, and amount of radiation protection to be installed in accordance with the final approved department layout and equipment selections. Where protected alcoves with view windows are required, a minimum of 1 foot 6 inches (0.45 meter) between the view window and the outside partition edge shall be provided. Radiation protection requirements shall be incorporated into the specifications and the building plans.

7.10.A3. Beds and stretchers shall have ready access to and from other departments of the institution. Particular attention should be paid to the management of outpatients for preparation and observation. The emergency, surgery, cystoscopy, and outpatient clinics should be accessible to the imaging suite. Imaging should be located on the ground floor, if practical, because of equipment ceiling height requirements, close proximity to electrical services, and expansion considerations.

7.10.A4. Flooring shall be adequate to meet load requirements for equipment, patients, and personnel. Provision for wiring raceways, ducts or conduits should be made in floors, walls, and ceilings. Ceiling heights may be higher than normal. Ceiling mounted equipment should have properly designed rigid support structures located above the finished ceiling. A lay-in type ceiling should be considered for ease of installation, service, and remodeling.

7.10.B. Angiography

7.10.B1. Space shall be provided as necessary to accommodate the functional program. The procedure room should be a minimum of 400 square feet (37.16 square meters).

7.10.B2. A control room shall be provided as necessary to meet the needs of the functional program. A view window shall be provided to permit full view of the patient.

7.10.B3. A viewing area shall be provided and should be a minimum of 10 feet (3.05 meters) in length.

7.10.B4. A scrub sink located outside the staff entry to the procedure room shall be provided for use by staff.

7.10.B5. A patient holding area should be provided to accommodate two stretchers with additional spaces for additional procedure rooms.

7.10.B6. Storage for portable equipment and catheters shall be provided.

7.10.B7. Provision shall be made within the facility for extended post-procedure observation of outpatients.

7.10.C. Computerized Tomography (CT) Scanning

7.10.C1. CT scan rooms shall be as required to accommodate the equipment.

7.10.C2. A control room shall be provided which is designed to accommodate the computer and other controls for the equipment. A view window shall be provided to permit full view of the patient. The angle between the control and equipment centroid shall permit the control operator to see the patient's head.

*7.10.C3. Computer room.

7.10.C4. The control room shall be located to allow convenient film processing.

7.10.C5. A patient toilet shall be provided. It shall be convenient to the procedure room, and if directly accessible to the scan room, arranged so that a patient may leave the toilet without having to reenter the scan room.

7.10.D. Diagnostic X-ray

*7.10.D1. Radiography rooms shall be of a size to accommodate the functional program.

*7.10.D2. Tomography, radiography/fluoroscopy rooms.

*7.10.D3. Mammography

7.10.D4. Each X-ray room shall include a shielded control alcove. This area shall be provided with a view window designed to provide full view of the examination table and the patient at all times, including full view of the patient when the table is in the tilt position or the chest X-ray is being utilized. For mammography machines with built-in shielding for the operator, the alcove may be omitted when approved by the certified physicist or state radiation protection agency.

7.10.E. Magnetic Resonance Imaging (MRI)

7.10.E1. Space shall be provided as necessary to accommodate the functional program. The MRI room may range from 325 square feet (30.22 square meters) to 620 square feet (57.66 square meters) depending on the vendor and magnet strength.

7.10.E2. A control room shall be provided with full view of the MRI and should be a minimum of 100 square feet (9.29 square meters), but may be larger depending on the vendor and magnet size.

7.10.E3. A computer room shall be provided and could range from 150 square feet (13.94 square meters) to 380 square feet (35.30 square meters) depending on the vendor and magnet strength. Self-contained air conditioning supplement is normally required.

*7.10.E4. Cryogen storage may be required in areas where service to replenish supplies is not readily available.

7.10.E5. A darkroom may be required for loading cassettes and shall be located near the control room. This darkroom shall be outside the 10-gauss field.

7.10.E6. When spectroscopy is provided, caution should be exercised in locating it in relation to the magnetic fringe fields.

7.10.E7. Power conditioning and voltage regulation equipment as well as direct current (DC) may be required.

7.10.E8. Magnetic shielding may be required to restrict the magnetic field plot. Radio frequency shielding is required to attenuate stray radio frequencies.

7.10.E9. A patient holding area should be located near the MRI unit and should be large enough to accommodate stretchers.

7.10.E10. Cryogen venting is required.

7.10.F. Ultrasound

7.10.F1. Space shall be provided as necessary to accommodate the functional program.

7.10.F2. A patient toilet, accessible from the procedure room and from the corridor, shall be provided.

7.10.G. Support Spaces

The following spaces are common to the imaging department and are minimum requirements unless stated otherwise:

7.10.G1. Patient Waiting Area

The area shall be out of traffic, under staff control, and shall have seating capacity in accordance with the functional program. If the suite is routinely used for outpatients and inpatients at the same time, separate waiting areas shall be provided with screening for visual privacy between the waiting areas.

If so determined by the hospital infection control risk assessment, the diagnostic imaging waiting area shall require special measures to reduce the risk of airborne infection transmission. These measures may included enhanced general ventilation and air disinfection techniques similar to inpatient requirements for airborne infection isolation rooms. See the CDC's "Guidelines for Preventing the Transmission of Mycobacterium Tuberculosis in Health Care Facilities."

7.10.G2. Control Desk and Reception Area

7.10.G3. Holding Area

A convenient holding area under staff control shall be provided to accommodate inpatients on stretchers or beds.

7.10.G4. Patient Toilet Rooms

Toilet rooms with handwashing facilities shall be provided convenient to the waiting rooms and shall be equipped with an emergency call system. Separate toilets with handwashing facilities shall be provided with direct access from each radiographic/fluoroscopic room so that a patient may leave the toilet without having to reenter the R&F room. Rooms used only occasionally for fluoroscopic procedures may utilize nearby patient toilets if they are located for immediate access.

7.10.G5. Patient Dressing Rooms

Dressing rooms shall be provided convenient to the waiting areas and X-ray rooms. Each room shall include a seat or bench, mirror, and provisions for hanging patients' clothing and for securing valuables.

7.10.G6. Staff Facilities

Toilets may be outside the suite but shall be convenient for staff use. In larger suites of three or more procedure rooms, toilets internal to the suite shall be provided. Staff lounge with lockers should be considered.

7.10.G7. Film Storage (Active)

A room with cabinet or shelves for filing patient film for immediate retrieval shall be provided.

7.10.G8. Film Storage (Inactive)

A room or area for inactive film storage shall be provided. It may be outside the imaging suite, but must be under imaging's administrative control and properly secured to protect films against loss or damage.

7.10.G9. Storage for Unexposed Film

Storage facilities for unexposed film shall include protection of film against exposure or damage and shall not be warmer than the air of adjacent occupied spaces.

7.10.G10. Offices for Radiologist(s) and Assistant(s)

Offices shall include provisions for viewing, individual consultation, and charting of film.

7.10.G11. Clerical Offices/Spaces

Office space shall be provided as necessary for the functional program.

7.10.G12. Consultation Area

An appropriate area for individual consultation with referring clinicians shall be provided.

7.10.G13. Contrast Media Preparation

This area shall be provided with sink, counter, and storage to allow for mixing of contrast media. One preparation room, if conveniently located, may serve any number of rooms. When preprepared media is used, this area may be omitted, but storage shall be provided for the media.

7.10.G14. Film Processing Room

A darkroom shall be provided for processing film unless the processing equipment normally used does not require a darkroom for loading and transfer. When daylight processing is used, the darkroom may be minimal for emergency and special uses. Film processing shall be located convenient to the procedure rooms and to the quality control area.

7.10.G15. Quality Control Area

An area or room shall be provided near the processor for viewing film immediately after it is processed. All view boxes shall be illuminated to provide light of the same color value and intensity for appropriate comparison of several adjacent films.

7.10.G16. Cleanup Facilities

Provisions for cleanup shall be located within the suite for convenient access and use. It shall include service sink or floor receptacle as well as storage space for equipment and supplies. If automatic film processors are used, a receptacle of adequate size with hot and cold water for cleaning the processor racks shall be provided.

7.10.G17. Handwashing Facilities

Handwashing facilities shall be provided within each procedure room unless the room is used only for routine screening such as chest X-rays where the patient is not physically handled by the staff. Handwashing facilities shall be provided convenient to the MRI room, but need not be within the room.

7.10.G18. Clean Storage

Provisions shall be made for the storage of clean supplies and linens. If conveniently located, storage may be shared with another department.

7.10.G19. Soiled Holding

Provisions shall be made for soiled holding. Separate provisions for contaminated handling and holding shall be made. Handwashing facilities shall be provided.

7.10.G20. Provision shall be made for locked storage of medications and drugs.

7.10.G21. Details and Finishes; Mechanical; Electrical
See Section 7.28 for details and finishes; 7.31 for mechanical; and 7.32 for electrical.

7.10.H. Cardiac Catheterization Lab (Cardiology)
Note: The number of procedure rooms and the size of the prep, holding, and recovery areas shall be based on expected utilization.

7.10.H1. The cardiac catheterization lab is normally a separate suite, but may be within the imaging suite provided that the appropriate sterile environment is provided. It can be combined with angiography in low usage situations.

7.10.H2. The procedure room shall be a minimum of 400 square feet (37.16 square meters) exclusive of fixed and movable cabinets and shelves.

7.10.H3. A control room or area shall be provided and shall be large enough to contain and provide for the efficient functioning of the X-ray and image recording equipment. A view window permitting full view of the patient from the control console shall be provided.

7.10.H4. An equipment room or enclosure large enough to contain X-ray transformers, power modules, and associated electronics and electrical gear shall be provided.

7.10.H5. Scrub facilities with hands-free operable controls shall be provided adjacent to the entrance of procedure rooms, and shall be arranged to minimize incidental splatter on nearby personnel, medical equipment, or supplies.

7.10.H6. Staff change area(s) shall be provided and arranged to ensure a traffic pattern so that personnel entering from outside the suite can enter, change their clothing, and move directly into the cardiac catheterization suite.

7.10.H7. A patient preparation, holding, and recovery area or room shall be provided and arranged to provide visual observation before and after the procedure.

7.10.H8. A clean workroom or clean supply room shall be provided. If the room is used for preparing patient care items, it shall contain a work counter and handwashing sink. If the room is used only for storage and holding of clean and sterile supply materials, the work counter and handwashing facilities may be omitted.

7.10.H9. A soiled workroom shall be provided which shall contain a handwashing and a clinical sink (or equivalent flushing rim fixtures). When the room is used for temporary holding or soiled materials, the clinical sink may be omitted.

7.10.H10. Housekeeping closet containing a floor receptor or service sink and provisions for storage of supplies and housekeeping equipment shall be provided.

7.10.H11. The following shall be available for use by the cardiac catheterization suite:

a. A viewing room.

b. A film file room.

7.11 Nuclear Medicine

7.11.A.
Equipment and space shall be provided as necessary to accommodate the functional program. Nuclear medicine may include positron emission tomography, which is not common to most facilities. It requires specialized planning for equipment.

7.11.B.
A certified physicist or other qualified expert representing the owner or state agency shall specify the type, location, and amount of radiation protection to be installed in accordance with final approved department layout and equipment selection. These specifications shall be incorporated into the plans.

7.11.C.
Flooring should meet load requirements for equipment, patients, and personnel. Floors and walls should be constructed of materials that are easily decontaminated in case of radioactive spills. Walls should contain necessary support systems for either built-in or mobile oxygen and vacuum, and vents for radioactive gases. Provision for wiring raceways, ducts, or conduits should be made in floors, walls, and ceilings. Ceilings may be higher than 8 feet (2.44 meters). Ceiling-mounted equipment should have properly designed rigid support structures located above the finished ceiling. A lay-in type ceiling should be considered for ease of service, installation, and remodeling.

7.11.D.
Space shall be provided as necessary to accommodate the functional program. When the functional program calls for it, the nuclear medicine room shall accommodate the equipment, a stretcher, exercise equipment (treadmill and/or bicycle), and staff.

7.11.E.
If radiopharmaceutical preparation is performed on-site, an area adequate to house a radiopharmacy shall be provided with appropriate shielding. This area should include adequate space for storage of radionuclides, chemicals for preparation, dose calibrators, and record-keeping. Floors and walls should be constructed of easily decontaminated materials. Vents and traps for radioactive gases should be provided if such are used. Hoods for

pharmaceutical preparation shall meet applicable standards. If pre-prepared materials are used, storage and calculation area may be considerably smaller than that for on-site preparation. Space shall provide adequately for dose calibration, quality assurance, and record keeping. The area may still require shielding from other portions of the facilities.

*7.11.F. Positron Emission Tomography (PET)

7.11.G.

Nuclear medicine area when operated separately from the imaging department shall include the following:

7.11.G1. Space shall be adequate to permit entry of stretchers, beds, and able to accommodate imaging equipment, electronic consoles, and if present, computer terminals.

7.11.G2. A darkroom on-site shall be available for film processing. The darkroom should contain protective storage facilities for unexposed film that guard the film against exposure or damage.

7.11.G3. When the functional program requires a centralized computer area, it should be a separate room with access terminals available within the imaging rooms.

7.11.G4. Provisions for cleanup shall be located within the suite for convenient access and use. It shall include service sink or floor receptacle as well as storage space for equipment and supplies.

7.11.G5. Film storage with cabinets or shelves for filing patient film for immediate retrieval shall be provided.

7.11.G6. Inactive film storage under the departmental administrative control and properly secured to protect film against loss or damage shall be provided.

7.11.G7. A consultation area with view boxes illuminated to provide light of the same color value and intensity for appropriate comparison of several adjacent films shall be provided. Space should be provided for computer access and display terminals if such are included in the program.

7.11.G8. Offices for physicians and assistants shall be provided and equipped for individual consultation, viewing, and charting of film.

7.11.G9. Clerical offices and spaces shall be provided as necessary for the program to function.

7.11.G10. Waiting areas shall be provided out of traffic, under staff control, and shall have seating capacity in accordance with the functional program. If the department is routinely used for outpatients and inpatients at the same time, separate waiting areas shall be provided with screening or visual privacy between the waiting areas.

7.11.G11. A dose administration area as specified by the functional program, shall be provided and located near the preparation area. Since as much as several hours may elapse for the dose to take effect, the area shall provide for visual privacy from other areas. Thought should be given to entertainment and reading materials.

7.11.G12. A holding area for patients on stretchers or beds shall be provided out of traffic and under control of staff and may be combined with the dose administration area with visual privacy between the areas.

7.11.G13. Patient dressing rooms shall be provided convenient to the waiting area and procedure rooms. Each dressing room shall include a seat or bench, a mirror, and provisions for hanging patients' clothing and for securing valuables.

7.11.G14. Toilet rooms shall be provided convenient to waiting and procedure rooms.

7.11.G15. Staff toilet(s) shall be provided convenient to the nuclear medicine laboratory.

7.11.G16. Handwashing facilities shall be provided within each procedure room.

7.11.G17. Control desk and reception area shall be provided.

7.11.G18. Storage area for clean linen with a handwashing facility shall be provided.

7.11.G19. Provisions with handwashing facilities shall be made for holding soiled material. Separate provisions shall be made for holding contaminated material.

7.11.G20. See Section 7.28 for details and finishes; 7.31 for mechanical; and 7.32 for electrical.

7.11.H. Radiotherapy Suite

7.11.H1. Rooms and spaces shall be provided as necessary to accommodate the functional program. Equipment manufacturers recommendations should be sought and followed, since space requirements may vary from one machine to another and one manufacturer to another. The radiotherapy suite may contain one or both electron beam therapy and radiation therapy. Although not recommended, a simulation room may be omitted in small linear accelerator facilities where other positioning geometry is provided.

7.11.H2. Cobalt, linear accelerators, and simulation rooms require radiation protection. A certified physicist representing the owner or appropriate state agency shall specify the type, location, and amount of protection to be installed in accordance with final approved department layout and equipment selection. The architect shall incorporate these specifications into the hospital building plans.

7.11.H3. Cobalt rooms and linear accelerators shall be sized in accordance with equipment requirements and shall accommodate a stretcher for litter-borne patients.

Layouts shall provide for preventing the escape of radioactive particles. Openings into the room, including doors, ductwork, vents, and electrical raceways and conduits, shall be baffled to prevent direct exposure to other areas of the facility.

*7.11.H4. Simulator, accelerator, and cobalt rooms shall be sized to accommodate the equipment with patient access on a stretcher, medical staff access to the equipment and patient, and service access.

7.11.H5. Flooring shall be adequate to meet load requirements for equipment, patients, and personnel. Provision for wiring raceways, ducts, or conduit should be made in floors and ceilings. Ceiling mounted equipment should have properly designed rigid support structures located above the finished ceiling. The ceiling height is normally higher than 8 feet (2.44 meters). A lay-in type of ceiling should be considered for ease of installation, service, and remodeling.

7.11.I. General Support Areas
The following areas shall be provided unless they are accessible from other areas such as imaging or OPD:

7.11.I1. A stretcher hold area adjacent to the treatment rooms, screened for privacy, and combined with a seating area for outpatients. The size of these areas will depend on the program for outpatients and inpatients.

7.11.I2. Exam rooms for each treatment room as specified by the functional program, each exam room to be a minimum of 100 square feet (9.29 square meters). Each exam room shall be equipped with a handwashing facility.

7.11.I3. Darkroom convenient to the treatment room(s) and the quality control area. Where daylight processing is used, the darkroom may be minimal for emergency use. If automatic film processors are used, a receptacle of adequate size with hot and cold water for cleaning the processor racks shall be provided either in the darkroom or nearby.

7.11.I4. Patient gowning area with provision for safe storage of valuables and clothing. At least one space should be large enough for staff-assisted dressing.

7.11.I5. Business office and/or reception/control area.

7.11.I6. Housekeeping room equipped with service sink or floor receptor and large enough for equipment or supplies storage.

7.11.I7. Film file area.

7.11.I8. Film storage area for unprocessed film.

7.11.J. Optional Support Areas
The following areas may be required by the functional program:

7.11.J1. Quality control area with view boxes illuminated to provide light of the same color value and intensity.

7.11.J2. Computer control area normally located just outside the entry to the treatment room(s).

7.11.J3. Dosimetry equipment area.

7.11.J4. Hypothermia room (may be combined with an exam room).

7.11.J5. Consultation room.

7.11.J6. Oncologist's office (may be combined with consultation room).

7.11.J7. Physicist's office (may be combined with treatment planning).

7.11.J8. Treatment planning and record room.

7.11.J9. Work station/nutrition station.

7.11.K. Additional Support Areas for Linear Accelerator:

7.11.K1. Mold room with exhaust hood and handwashing facility.

7.11.K2. Block room with storage. The block room may be combined with the mold room.

7.11.L. Additional Support Areas for Cobalt Room:

7.11.L1. Hot lab.

7.12 Laboratory Suite

Laboratory facilities shall be provided for the performance of tests in hematology, clinical chemistry, urinalysis, microbiology, anatomic pathology, cytology, and blood banking to meet the workload described in the functional program. Certain procedures may be performed on-site or provided through a contractual arrangement with a laboratory service acceptable to the authority having local jurisdiction.

Provisions shall be made for the following procedures to be performed on-site: blood counts, urinalysis, blood glucose, electrolytes, blood urea and nitrogen (BUN), coagulation, and transfusions (type and cross-match capability). Provisions shall also be included for specimen collection and processing.

The following physical facilities shall be provided within the hospital:

7.12.A.
Laboratory work counter(s) with space for microscopes, appropriate chemical analyzer(s), incubator(s), centrifuge(s), etc. shall be provided. Work areas shall include sinks with water and access to vacuum, gases, and air, and electrical services as needed.

7.12.B.

Refrigerated blood storage facilities for transfusions shall be provided. Blood storage refrigerator shall be equipped with temperature-monitoring and alarm signals.

7.12.C.

Lavatory(ies) or counter sink(s) equipped for handwashing shall be provided. Counter sinks may also be used for disposal of nontoxic fluids.

*7.12.D.

Storage facilities, including refrigeration, for reagents, standards, supplies, and stained specimen microscope slides, etc. shall be provided. Such facilities shall conform to applicable NFPA standards.

7.12.E.

Specimen (blood, urine, and feces) collection facility shall be provided. Blood collection area shall have work counter, space for patient seating, and handwashing facilities. Urine and feces collection room shall be equipped with water closet and lavatory. This facility may be located outside the laboratory suite.

7.12.F.

Chemical safety provisions including emergency shower, eyeflushing devices, and appropriate storage for flammable liquids, etc., shall be made.

7.12.G.

Facilities and equipment for terminal sterilization of contaminated specimens before transport (autoclave or electric oven) shall be provided. (Terminal sterilization is not required for specimens that are incinerated on-site.)

7.12.H.

If radioactive materials are employed, facilities shall be available for long-term storage and disposal of these materials. No special provisions will normally be required for body waste products from most patients receiving low level isotope diagnostic material. Requirements of authorities having jurisdiction should be verified.

7.12.I.

Administrative areas including offices as well as space for clerical work, filing, and record maintenance shall be provided.

7.12.J.

Lounge, locker, and toilet facilities shall be conveniently located for male and female laboratory staff. These may be outside the laboratory area and shared with other departments.

The functional program shall describe the type and location of all special equipment that is to be wired, plumbed, or plugged in, and the utilities required to operate each.

Note: Refer to NFPA code requirements applicable to hospital laboratories, including standards clarifying that hospital units do not necessarily have the same fire safety requirements as commercial chemical laboratories.

7.13 Rehabilitation Therapy Department

7.13.A. General

Rehabilitation therapy is primarily for restoration of body functions and may contain one or several categories of services. If a formal rehabilitative therapy service is included in a project, the facilities and equipment shall be as necessary for the effective function of the program. When two or more rehabilitative services are included, items may be shared, as appropriate.

7.13.B. Common Elements

Each rehabilitative therapy department shall include the following, which may be shared or provided as separate units for each service:

7.13.B1. Office and clerical space with provision for filing and retrieval of patient records.

7.13.B2. Reception and control station(s) with visual control of waiting and activities areas. (This may be combined with office and clerical space.)

7.13.B3. Patient waiting area(s) out of traffic with provision for wheelchairs.

7.13.B4. Patient toilets with handwashing facilities accessible to wheelchair patients.

7.13.B5. Space(s) for storing wheelchairs and stretchers out of traffic while patients are using the services. These spaces may be separate from the service area but must be conveniently located.

7.13.B6. A conveniently accessible housekeeping room and service sink for housekeeping use.

7.13.B7. Locking closets or cabinets within the vicinity of each work area for securing staff personal effects.

7.13.B8. Convenient access to toilets and lockers.

7.13.B9. Access to a demonstration/conference room.

7.13.C. Physical Therapy

If physical therapy is part of the service, the following, at least, shall be included:

7.13.C1. Individual treatment area(s) with privacy screens or curtains. Each such space shall have not less than 70 square feet (6.51 square meters) of clear floor area.

7.13.C2. Handwashing facilities for staff either within or at each treatment space. (One handwashing facility may serve several treatment stations.)

7.13.C3. Exercise area and facilities.

7.13.C4. Clean linen and towel storage.

7.13.C5. Storage for equipment and supplies.

7.13.C6. Separate storage for soiled linen, towels, and supplies.

7.13.C7. If required by the functional program, patient dressing areas, showers, and lockers. These shall be accessible and usable by the disabled.

7.13.C8. Provisions shall be made for thermotherapy, diathermy, ultrasonics, and hydrotherapy when required by the functional program.

7.13.D. Occupational Therapy
If this service is provided, the following, at least, shall be included:

7.13.D1. Work areas and counters suitable for wheelchair access.

7.13.D2. Handwashing facilities.

7.13.D3. Storage for supplies and equipment.

*7.13.D4. An area for teaching daily living activities shall be provided. It shall contain an area for a bed, kitchen counter with appliances and sink, bathroom, and a table/chair.

7.13.E. Prosthetics and Orthotics
If this service is provided, the following, at least, shall be included:

7.13.E1. Work space for technicians

7.13.E2. Space for evaluating and fitting, with provision for privacy.

7.13.E3. Space for equipment, supplies, and storage.

7.13.F. Speech and Hearing
If this service is provided, the following, at least, shall be included:

7.13.F1. Space for evaluation and treatment.

7.13.F2. Space for equipment and storage.

7.14 Renal Dialysis Unit (Acute and Chronic)

7.14.A. General

7.14.A1. The number of dialysis stations shall be based upon the expected workload and may include several work shifts per day.

7.14.A2. The location shall offer convenient access for outpatients. Accessibility to the unit from parking and public transportation shall be a consideration.

7.14.A3. Space and equipment shall be provided as necessary to accommodate the functional programs which may include acute (inpatient services) and chronic cases, home treatment and kidney reuse facilities. Inpatient services (acute) may be performed in critical care units and designated areas in the hospital, with appropriate utility.

7.14.B. Treatment Area

7.14.B1. The treatment area may be an open area and shall be separate from administrative and waiting areas.

7.14.B2. Nurses' station(s) shall be located within the dialysis treatment area and designed to provide visual observation of all patient stations.

7.14.B3. Individual patient treatment areas shall contain at least 80 square feet (7.43 square meters). There shall be at least a 4-foot (1.22 meters) space between beds and/or lounge chairs.

7.14.B4. Handwashing facilities shall be convenient to the nurses station and patient treatment areas. There shall be at least one handwashing facility serving no more than four stations. These shall be uniformly distributed to provide equal access from each patient station.

7.14.B5. The open unit shall be designed to provide privacy for each patient.

7.14.B6. The number of and need for required airborne infection isolation rooms shall be determined by an infection control risk assessment. When required, the airborne infection isolation room(s) shall comply with the requirements of Section 7.2.C.

7.14.B7. If required by the functional program, there shall be a medication dispensing station for the dialysis center. A work counter and handwashing facilities shall be included in this area. Provisions shall be made for the controlled storage, preparation distribution and refrigeration of medications.

7.14.B8. If home training is provided in the unit, a private treatment area of at least 120 square feet (11.15 square meters) shall be provided for patients who are being trained to use dialysis equipment at home. This room shall contain counter, handwashing facilities, and a separate drain for fluid disposal.

7.14.B9. An examination room with handwashing facilities and writing surface shall be provided with at least 100 square feet (9.29 square meters).

7.14.B10. A clean workroom shall be provided. If the room is used for preparing patient care items, it shall contain a work counter, a handwashing facility, and storage facilities for clean and sterile supplies. If the room is used only for storage and holding as part of a system for distribution of clean and sterile materials, the work counter and handwashing facility may be omitted. Soiled and clean workrooms or holding rooms shall be separated and have no direct connection.

7.14.B11. A soiled workroom shall be provided and contain a flushing-rim sink, handwashing sink, work counter, storage cabinets, waste receptacles and a soiled linen receptacle.

7.14.B12. If dialyzers are reused, a reprocessing room is required, sized to perform the functions required and to include one-way flow of materials from soiled to clean with provisions for a refrigeration (temporary storage or dialyzer) decontamination/cleaning areas, sinks processors, computer processors and label printers, packaging area and dialyzer storage cabinets.

7.14.B13. If a nourishment station for the dialysis service is provided, the nourishment station shall contain a sink, a work counter, a refrigerator, storage cabinets and equipment for serving nourishments as required.

7.14.B14. An environmental services closet shall be provided adjacent to and for the exclusive use of the unit. The closet shall contain a floor receptor or service sink and storage space for housekeeping supplies and equipment.

7.14.B15. If required by the functional program, an equipment repair and breakdown room shall be equipped with a handwashing facility, deep service sink, work counter and storage cabinet.

7.14.B16. Supply areas or supply carts shall be provided.

7.14.B17. Storage space shall be available for wheelchairs and stretchers, if stretchers are provided, out of direct line of traffic.

7.14.B18. A clean linen storage area shall be provided. This may be within the clean workroom, a separate closet, or an approved distribution system. If a closed cart system is used, storage may be in an alcove. It must be out of the path of normal traffic and under staff control.

7.14.B19. Each facility using a central batch delivery system shall provide, either on the premises or through written arrangements, individual delivery systems for the treatment of any patient requiring special dialysis solutions. The mixing room should also include a sink, storage space and holding tanks.

7.14.B20. The water treatment equipment shall be located in an enclosed room.

7.14.B21. A patient toilet with handwashing facilities shall be provided.

7.14.C. Ancillary Facilities

7.14.C1. Appropriate areas shall be available for male and female personnel for staff clothing change area and lounge. The areas shall contain lockers, shower, toilet, and handwashing facilities.

7.14.C2. Storage for patients' belongings shall be provided.

7.14.C3. A waiting room, toilet room with handwashing facilities, drinking fountain, public telephone, and seating accommodations for waiting periods shall be available or accessible to the dialysis unit.

7.14.C4. Office and clinical work space shall be available for administrative services.

7.15 Respiratory Therapy Service

The type and extent of respiratory therapy service in different institutions vary greatly. In some, therapy is delivered in large sophisticated units, centralized in a specific area; in others, basic services are provided only at patients' bedsides. If respiratory service is provided, the following elements shall be included as a minimum, in addition to those elements stipulated in Sections 7.13B1, 7, 8, and 9:

7.15.A. Storage for Equipment and Supplies

7.15.B.
Space and Utilities for Cleaning and Disinfecting Equipment. Provide physical separation of the space for receiving and cleaning soiled materials from the space for storage of clean equipment and supplies. Appropriate local exhaust ventilation shall be provided if glutaraldehyde or other noxious disinfectants are used in the cleaning process.

7.15.C.
Respiratory services shall be conveniently accessible on a 24-hour basis to the critical care units.

7.15.D.
If respiratory services such as testing and demonstration for outpatients are part of the program, additional facilities and equipment shall be provided as necessary for the appropriate function of the service, including but not limited to:

7.15.D1. Patient waiting area with provision for wheelchairs.

7.15.D2. A reception and control station.

7.15.D3. Patient toilets and handwashing facilities.

7.15.D4. Room(s) for patient education and demonstration.

7.15.E. Cough-Inducing and Aerosol-Generating Procedures

All cough-inducing procedures performed on patients who may have infectious *Mycobacterium tuberculosis* shall be performed in rooms using local exhaust ventilation devices, e.g., booths or special enclosures with discharge HEPA filters and exhaust directly to the outside. These procedures may also be performed in a room that meets the ventilation requirements for noxious gas or airborne infection control. See Table 2 for ventilation requirements.

7.16 Morgue

These facilities shall be accessible through an exterior entrance and shall be located to avoid the need for transporting bodies through public areas.

7.16.A.
The following elements shall be provided when autopsies are performed in the hospital:

7.16.A1. Refrigerated facilities for body holding.

7.16.A2. An autopsy room containing the following:

a. A work counter with a sink equipped for handwashing.

b. A storage space for supplies, equipment, and specimens.

c. An autopsy table.

d. A deep sink for washing of specimens.

7.16.A3. A housekeeping service sink or receptor for cleanup and housekeeping.

*7.16.B.
If autopsies are performed outside the facility, a well-ventilated, temperature-controlled, body-holding room shall be provided.

7.17 Pharmacy

7.17.A. General
The size and type of services to be provided in the pharmacy will depend upon the type of drug distribution system used, number of patients to be served, and extent of shared or purchased services. This shall be described in the functional program. The pharmacy room or suite shall be located for convenient access, staff control, and security. Facilities and equipment shall be as necessary to accommodate the functions of the program. (Satellite facilities, if provided, shall include those items required by the program.) As a minimum, the following elements shall be included:

7.17.B. Dispensing

7.17.B1. A pickup and receiving area.

7.17.B2. An area for reviewing and recording.

7.17.B3. An extemporaneous compounding area that includes a sink and sufficient counter space for drug preparation. Floor drainage may also be required, depending on the extent of compounding conducted.

7.17.B4. Work counters and space for automated and manual dispensing activities.

7.17.B5. An area for temporary storage, exchange, and restocking of carts.

7.17.B6. Security provisions for drugs and personnel in the dispensing counter area.

7.17.C. Manufacturing

7.17.C1. A bulk compounding area.

7.17.C2. Provisions for packaging and labeling.

7.17.C3. A quality-control area.

7.17.D. Storage (may be cabinets, shelves, and/or separate rooms or closets)

7.17.D1. Bulk storage.

7.17.D2. Active storage.

7.17.D3. Refrigerated storage.

7.17.D4. Volatile fluids and alcohol storage constructed according to applicable fire safety codes for the substances involved.

7.17.D5. Secure storage for narcotics and controlled drugs.

7.17.D6. Storage for general supplies and equipment not in use.

7.17.E. Administration

7.17.E1. Provision for cross-checking of medication and drug profiles of individual patients.

7.17.E2. Poison control, reaction data, and drug information centers.

7.17.E3. A separate room or area for office function including desk, filing, communication, and reference.

7.17.E4. Provisions for patient counseling and instruction (may be in a room separate from the pharmacy).

7.17.E5. A room for education and training (may be in a multipurpose room shared with other departments).

7.17.F. Other

7.17.F1. Handwashing facilities shall be provided within each separate room where open medication is handled.

7.17.F2. Provide for convenient access to toilet and locker.

7.17.F3. If unit dose procedure is used, provide additional space and equipment for supplies, packaging, labeling, and storage, as well as for the carts.

7.17.F4. If IV solutions are prepared in the pharmacy, provide a sterile work area with a laminar-flow workstation designed for product protection. The laminar-flow system shall include a nonhydroscopic filter rated at 99.97 percent (HEPA), as tested by DOP tests, and have a visible pressure gauge for detection of filter leaks or defects.

7.17.F5. Provide for consultation and patient education when the functional program requires dispensing of medication to outpatients.

7.18 Dietary Facilities

7.18.A. General
Food service facilities and equipment shall conform with these standards and with the standards of the National Sanitation Foundation and other appropriate codes and shall provide food service for staff, visitors, inpatients, and outpatients as may be appropriate.

Consideration may also be required for meals to VIP suites, and for cafeterias for staff, ambulatory patients, and visitors as well as providing for nourishments and snacks between scheduled meal service.

Patient food preparation areas shall be located in an area adjacent to delivery, interior transportation, storage, etc.

Finishes in the dietary facility shall be selected to ensure cleanability and the maintenance of sanitary conditions.

7.18.B. Functional Elements
If on-site conventional food service preparation is used, the following shall be provided in size and number appropriate for the approved function:

7.18.B1. Receiving/control stations. Provide an area for the receiving and control of incoming dietary supplies. This area shall be separated from the general receiving area and shall contain the following: a control station and a breakout for loading, uncrating, and weighing supplies.

7.18.B2. Storage spaces. They shall be convenient to the receiving area and shall be located to exclude traffic through the food preparation area to reach them. Storage spaces for bulk, refrigerated, and frozen foods shall be provided. A minimum of four days' supplies shall be stocked. (In remote areas, this number may be increased to accommodate length of delivery in emergencies.)

Food storage components shall be grouped for convenient access from receiving and to the food preparation areas.

All food shall be stored clear of the floor. Lowest shelf shall be not less than 12 inches (30 centimeters) above the floor or shall be closed in and sealed tight for ease of cleaning.

7.18.B3. Cleaning supplies storage. Provide a separate storage room for the storage of nonfood items such as cleaning supplies that might contaminate edibles.

7.18.B4. Additional storage rooms. They shall be provided as necessary for the storage of cooking wares, extra trays, flatware, plastic and paper products, and portable equipment.

7.18.B5. Food preparation work spaces. Provide work spaces for food preparation, cooking, and baking. These areas shall be as close as possible to the user (i.e., tray assembly and dining). Provide additional spaces for thawing and portioning.

7.18.B6. Assembly and distribution. Provide a patient tray assembly area and locate within close proximity to the food preparation and distribution areas.

7.18.B7. Food service carts. A cart distribution system shall be provided with spaces for storage, loading, distribution, receiving, and sanitizing of the food service carts. The cart traffic shall be designed to eliminate any danger of cross-circulation between outgoing food carts and incoming, soiled carts, and the cleaning and sanitizing process. Cart circulation shall not be through food processing areas.

7.18.B8. Dining area. Provide dining space(s) for ambulatory patients, staff, and visitors. These spaces shall be separate from the food preparation and distribution areas.

7.18.B9. Vending services. If vending devices are used for unscheduled meals, provide a separate room that can be accessed without having to enter the main dining area. The vending room shall contain coin-operated machines, bill changers, a handwashing fixture, and a sitting area. Facilities for the servicing and sanitizing of the machines shall be provided as part of the food service program of the facility.

7.18.B10. Area for receiving, scraping, and sorting soiled tableware shall be adjacent to ware washing and separate from food preparation areas.

7.18.B11. Ware washing facilities. They shall be designed to prevent contamination of clean wares with soiled wares through cross-traffic. The clean wares shall be transferred for storage or use in the dining area without having to pass through food preparation areas.

7.18.B12. Pot washing facilities including multi-compartmented sinks of adequate size for intended use shall be provided convenient to using service. Supplemental heat for hot water to clean pots and pans may be by booster heater or by steam jet.

Mobile carts or other provisions should be made for drying and storage of pots and pans.

7.18.B13. Waste storage room. A food waste storage room shall be conveniently located to the food preparation and ware washing areas but not within the food preparation area. It shall have direct access to the hospital's waste collection and disposal facilities.

7.18.B14. Handwashing. Fixtures that are operable without the use of hands shall be located conveniently accessible at locations throughout the unit.

7.18.B15. Office spaces. Offices for the use of the food service manager shall be provided. In smaller facilities, this space may be located in an area that is part of the food preparation area.

7.18.B16. Toilets and locker spaces. Spaces shall be provided for the exclusive use of the dietary staff. They shall not open directly into the food preparation areas, but must be in close proximity to them.

7.18.B17. Housekeeping rooms. They shall be provided for the exclusive use of the dietary department and shall contain the following: a floor sink and space for mops, pails, and supplies. Where hot water or steam is used for general cleaning, additional space within the room shall be provided for the storage of hoses and nozzles.

7.18.B18. Icemaking equipment. It shall be of type that is convenient for service and easily cleaned. It shall be provided for both drinks and food products (self-dispensing equipment) and for general use (storage-bin type equipment).

7.18.B19. Commissary or contract services from other areas. Items above may be reduced as appropriate. Provide for protection of food delivered to insure freshness, retention of hot and cold, and avoidance of contamination. If delivery is from outside sources, provide protection against weather. Provisions must be made for thorough cleaning and sanitizing of equipment to avoid mix of soiled and clean.

7.18.C. Equipment
Mechanical devices shall be heavy duty, suitable for use intended, and easily cleaned. Where equipment is movable provide heavy duty locking casters. If equipment is to have fixed utility connections, the equipment should not be equipped with casters. Walk-in coolers, refrigerators, and freezers shall be insulated at floor as well as at walls and top. Coolers and refrigerators shall be capable of maintaining a temperature down to freezing. Freezers shall be capable of maintaining a temperature of 20

degrees below 0 F. Coolers, refrigerators, and freezers shall be thermostatically controlled to maintain desired temperature settings in increments of 2 degrees or less. Interior temperatures shall be indicated digitally so as to be visible from the exterior. Controls shall include audible and visible high and low temperature alarm. Time of alarm shall be automatically recorded.

Walk-in units may be lockable from outside but must have a release mechanism for exit from inside at all times. Interior shall be lighted. All shelving shall be corrosion resistant, easily cleaned, and constructed and anchored to support a loading of at least 100 pounds per linear foot.

All cooking equipment shall be equipped with automatic shut-off devices to prevent excessive heat buildup.

Under-counter conduits, piping, and drains shall be arranged to not interfere with cleaning of floor below or of the equipment.

7.19 Administration and Public Areas

The following shall be provided:

7.19.A. Entrance
This shall be at grade level, sheltered from inclement weather, and accessible to the disabled.

7.19.B. Lobby
This shall include:

7.19.B1. A counter or desk for reception and information.

7.19.B2. Public waiting area(s).

7.19.B3. Public toilet facilities.

7.19.B4. Public telephones.

7.19.B5. Drinking fountain(s).

7.19.C. Interview Space(s)
These shall include provisions for private interviews relating to social service, credit, and admissions.

7.19.D. Admissions Area
If required by the functional program for initial admission of inpatients, the area shall include:

7.19.D1. A separate waiting area for patients and accompanying persons.

7.19.D2. A work counter or desk for staff.

7.19.D3. A storage area for wheelchairs, out of the path of normal traffic.

7.19.E. General or Individual Office(s)
These shall be provided for business transactions, medical and financial records, and administrative and professional staff.

7.19.F. Multipurpose Room(s)

These shall be provided for conferences, meetings, and health education purposes, and include provisions for the use of visual aids. One multipurpose room may be shared by several services.

7.19.G. Storage for Office Equipment and Supplies

7.20 Medical Records

Rooms, areas, or offices for the following personnel and/or functions shall be provided:

7.20.A. Medical Records Administrator/Technician

7.20.B. Review and Dictation

7.20.C. Sorting, Recording, or Microfilming Records

7.20.D. Record Storage

7.21 Central Services

The following shall be provided:

7.21.A. Separate Soiled and Clean Work Areas

7.21.A1. Soiled workroom
This room shall be physically separated from all other areas of the department. Work space should be provided to handle the cleaning and initial sterilization/disinfection of all medical/surgical instruments and equipment, work tables, sinks, flush-type devices, and washer/sterilizer decontaminators. Pass-through doors and washer/sterilizer decontaminators should deliver into clean processing area/workrooms.

*7.21.A2. Clean Assembly/Workroom
This workroom shall contain handwashing facilities, workspace, and equipment for terminal sterilizing of medical and surgical equipment and supplies. Clean and soiled work areas should be physically separated.

7.21.B. Storage Areas

7.21.B1. Clean/Sterile Medical/Surgical Supplies
A room for breakdown should be provided for manufacturers' clean/sterile supplies (clean processing area should not be in this area but adjacent). Storage for packs etc., shall include provisions for ventilation, humidity, and temperature control.

7.21.C. Administrative/Changing Room

If required by the functional program, this room should be separate from all other areas and provide for staff to change from street clothes into work attire. Lockers, sink, and showers should be made available within the immediate vicinity of the department.

7.21.D. Storage Room for Patient Care and Distribution Carts

This area should be adjacent, easily available to clean and sterile storage, and close to main distribution point to keep traffic to a minimum and to ease work flow.

7.22 General Stores

In addition to supply facilities in individual departments, a central storage area shall also be provided. General stores may be located in a separate building on-site with provisions for protection against inclement weather during transfer of supplies.

The following shall be provided:

7.22.A. Off-street Unloading Facilities

7.22.B. Receiving Area

7.22.C. General Storage Room(s)

General storage room(s) with a total area of not less than 20 square feet (1.86 square meters) per inpatient bed shall be provided. Storage may be in separate, concentrated areas within the institution or in one or more individual buildings on-site. A portion of this storage may be provided off-site.

7.22.D. Additional Storage Room(s)

Additional storage areas for outpatient facilities shall be provided in an amount not less than 5 percent of the total area of the outpatient facilities. This may be combined with and in addition to the general stores or be located in a central area within the outpatient department. A portion of this storage may be provided off-site.

7.23 Linen Services

7.23.A. General

Each facility shall have provisions for storing and processing of clean and soiled linen for appropriate patient care. Processing may be done within the facility, in a separate building on- or off-site, or in a commercial or shared laundry.

7.23.B.

Facilities and equipment shall be as required for cost effective operation as described in the functional program. At a minimum, the following elements shall be included:

7.23.B1. A separate room for receiving and holding soiled linen until ready for pickup or processing.

7.23.B2. A central, clean linen storage and issuing room(s), in addition to the linen storage required at individual patient units.

7.23.B3. Cart storage area(s) for separate parking of clean- and soiled-linen carts out of traffic.

7.23.B4. A clean linen inspection and mending room or area. If not provided elsewhere, a clean linen inspection, delinting, folding, assembly, and packaging area should be provided as part of the linen services. Mending should be provided for in the linen services department. A space for tables, shelving, and storage should be provided.

7.23.B5. Handwashing facilities in each area where unbagged, soiled linen is handled.

7.23.C.
If linen is processed outside the building, provisions shall also be made for:

7.23.C1. A service entrance, protected from inclement weather, for loading and unloading of linen.

7.23.C2. Control station for pickup and receiving.

7.23.D.
If linen is processed in a laundry facility that is part of the project (within or as a separate building), the following shall be provided in addition to that of Section 7.23.B:

7.23.D1. A receiving, holding, and sorting room for control and distribution of soiled linen. Discharge from soiled linen chutes may be received within this room or in a separate room.

7.23.D2. Laundry processing room with commercial type equipment that can process at least a seven-day supply within the regular scheduled work week. This may require a capacity for processing a seven-day supply in a 40-hour week.

7.23.D3. Storage for laundry supplies.

7.23.D4. Employee handwashing facilities in each room where clean or soiled linen is processed and handled.

7.23.D5. Arrangement of equipment that will permit an orderly work flow and minimize cross-traffic that might mix clean and soiled operations.

7.23.D6. Conveniently accessible staff lockers, showers, and lounge.

7.24 Facilities for Cleaning and Sanitizing Carts

Facilities shall be provided to clean and sanitize carts serving the central service department, dietary facilities, and linen services. These facilities may be centralized or departmentalized.

7.25 Employee Facilities

Lockers, lounges, toilets, etc. should be provided for employees and volunteers. These should be in addition to, and separate from, those required for medical staff and public.

7.26 Housekeeping Rooms

In addition to the housekeeping rooms required in certain departments, sufficient housekeeping rooms shall be provided throughout the facility as required to maintain a clean and sanitary environment. Each shall contain a floor receptor or service sink and storage space for housekeeping equipment and supplies. There shall not be less than one housekeeping room for each floor.

7.27 Engineering Service and Equipment Areas

Sufficient space shall be included in all mechanical and electrical equipment rooms for proper maintenance of equipment. Provisions shall also be made for removal and replacement of equipment.

7.27.A.
Room(s) or separate building(s) for boilers, mechanical, and electrical equipment, except:

7.27.A1. Roof-top air conditioning and ventilation equipment installed in weatherproof housings.

7.27.A2. Standby generators where the engine and appropriate accessories (e.g., batteries) are properly heated and enclosed in a weatherproof housing.

7.27.A3. Cooling towers and heat rejection equipment.

7.27.A4. Electrical transformers and switchgear where required to serve the facility and where installed in a weatherproof housing.

7.27.A5. Medical gas parks and equipment.

7.27.A6. Air-cooled chillers where installed in a weatherproof housing.

7.27.A7. Trash compactors and incinerators. Site lighting, post indicator valves, and other equipment normally installed on the exterior of the building.

7.27.B.
Engineer's office with file space and provisions for protected storage of facility drawings, records, manuals, etc.

7.27.C.
General maintenance shop(s) for repair and maintenance.

7.27.D.

Storage room for building maintenance supplies. Storage for solvents and flammable liquids shall comply with applicable NFPA codes.

7.27.E.

Separate area or room specifically for storage, repair, and testing of electronic and other medical equipment. The amount of space and type of utilities will vary with the type of equipment involved and types of outside contracts used.

7.27.F.

Yard equipment and supply storage areas shall be located so that equipment may be moved directly to the exterior without interference with other work.

7.28 General Standards for Details and Finishes

If approved by the authorities having jurisdiction, retained portions of existing facilities that are not required to be totally modernized due to financial or other hardships may, as a minimum, comply with applicable requirements of the Existing Health Care Occupancies Section of NFPA 101. However, a plan of correction for these portions should also be developed and implemented.

Details and finishes in new construction projects, including additions and alterations, shall comply with the following (see Section 1.2 concerning existing facilities where total compliance is structurally impractical):

7.28.A. Details

7.28.A1. Compartmentation, exits, fire alarms, automatic extinguishing systems, and other fire prevention and fire protection measures, including those within existing facilities, shall comply with NFPA 101, with the following stipulation. The Fire-Safety Evaluation System (FSES) shall not be used as a substitute for basic NFPA 101 design criteria for new construction or major renovations in existing facilities. (The FSES is intended as an evaluation tool for fire safety only.) See Section 1.5 for exceptions. Note: For most projects it is essential that third-party reimbursement requirements also be followed. Verify where these may be in excess of standards in these Guidelines.

7.28.A2. Corridors in outpatient suites and in areas not commonly used for patient bed or stretcher transportation may be reduced in width to 5 feet (1.52 meters).

7.28.A3. Location of items such as drinking fountains, telephone booths, vending machines, and portable equipment shall not restrict corridor traffic or reduce the corridor width below the minimum standard.

7.28.A4. Rooms that contain bathtubs, sitz baths, showers, and/or water closets for inpatient use shall be equipped with doors and hardware permitting emergency access from the outside. When such rooms have only one opening or are small, the doors shall open outward or in a manner that will avoid pressing a patient who may have collapsed within the room. Similar considerations may be desirable for certain outpatient services.

7.28.A5. If required by the program, door hardware on patient toilet rooms in psychiatric nursing units may be designed to allow staff to control access.

7.28.A6. The minimum door size for inpatient bedrooms in new work shall be 3 feet 8 inches (1.12 meters) wide and 7 feet (2.13 meters) high to provide clearance for movement of beds and other equipment. Existing doors of not less than 2 feet 10 inches (86.36 centimeters) wide may be considered for acceptance where function is not adversely affected and replacement is impractical. Doors to other rooms used for stretchers (including hospital wheeled-bed stretchers) and/or wheelchairs shall have a minimum width of 2 feet 10 inches (86.36 centimeters). Where used in these Guidelines, door width and height shall be the nominal dimension of the door leaf, ignoring projections of frame and stops. **Note:** While these standards are intended for access by patients and patient equipment, size of office furniture, etc., shall also be considered.

7.28.A7. All doors between corridors, rooms, or spaces subject to occupancy, except elevator doors, shall be of the swing type. Manual or automatic sliding doors may be exempt from this standard where fire and other emergency exiting requirements are not compromised and where cleanliness of surfaces can be maintained.

7.28.A8. Doors, except those to spaces such as small closets not subject to occupancy, shall not swing into corridors in a manner that might obstruct traffic flow or reduce the required corridor width. (Large walk-in-type closets are considered inhabitable spaces.)

7.28.A9. Windows and outer doors that frequently may be left open shall be equipped with insect screens.

7.28.A10. Patient rooms or suites in new construction intended for 24-hour occupancy shall have windows or vents that can be opened from the inside to vent noxious fumes and smoke products and to bring in fresh air in emergencies. Operation of such windows shall be restricted to inhibit possible escape or suicide. Where the operation of windows or vents requires the use of tools or keys, these shall be on the same floor and easily accessible to staff. Windows in existing buildings designed with approved engineered smoke-control systems may be of fixed construction.

7.28.A11. Glass doors, lights, sidelights, borrowed lights, and windows located within 12 inches (30 centimeters) of a door jamb (with a bottom-frame height of less than 60 inches or 1.52 meters above the finished floor) shall be constructed of safety glass, wired glass, or plastic, break-resistant material that creates no dangerous cutting edges when broken. Similar materials shall be used for wall openings in active areas such as recreation and exercise rooms, unless otherwise required for fire safety. Safety glass-tempered or plastic glazing materials shall be used for shower doors and bath enclosures. Plastic and similar materials used for glazing shall comply with the flame-spread ratings of NFPA 101. Safety glass or plastic glazing materials, as noted above, shall also be used for interior windows and doors, including those in pediatric and psychiatric unit corridors. In renovation projects, only glazing within 18 inches (46 centimeters) of the floor must be changed to safety glass, wire glass, or plastic, break-resistant material.

Note: Provisions of this paragraph concern safety from hazards of breakage. NFPA 101 contains additional requirements for glazing in exit corridors, etc., especially in buildings without sprinkler systems.

7.28.A12. Linen and refuse chutes shall meet or exceed the following standards:

a. Service openings to chutes shall comply with NFPA 101.

b. The minimum cross-sectional dimension of gravity chutes shall be 2 feet (60.96 centimeters).

c. Chute discharge into collection rooms shall comply with NFPA 101.

d. Chutes shall meet the provisions as described in NFPA 82.

7.28.A13. Thresholds and expansion joint covers shall be flush with the floor surface to facilitate the use of wheelchairs and carts. Expansion and seismic joints shall be constructed to restrict the passage of smoke.

7.28.A14. Grab bars shall be provided in all patient toilets, showers, bathtubs, and sitz baths at a wall clearance of 1½ inches (3.81 centimeters). Bars, including those which are part of such fixtures as soap dishes, shall be sufficiently anchored to sustain a concentrated load of 250 pounds (113.4 kilograms).

7.28.A15. Location and arrangement of fittings for handwashing facilities shall permit their proper use and operation. Particular care should be given to the clearances required for blade-type operating handles.

7.28.A16. Mirrors shall not be installed at handwashing fixtures in food preparation areas, nurseries, clean and sterile supply areas, scrub sinks, or other areas where asepsis control would be lessened by hair combing.

7.28.A17. Provisions for hand drying shall be included at all handwashing facilities except scrub sinks. These provisions shall be paper or cloth units enclosed to protect against dust or soil and to insure single-unit dispensing. Hot air dryers are permitted provided that installation precludes possible contamination by recirculation of air.

7.28.A18. Lavatories and handwashing facilities shall be securely anchored to withstand an applied vertical load of not less than 250 pounds (113.4 kilograms) on the fixture front.

7.28.A19. Radiation protection requirements for X-ray and gamma ray installations shall conform with NCRP Report Nos. 33 and 49 and all applicable local requirements. Provision shall be made for testing completed installations before use. All defects must be corrected before approval. Testing is to be coordinated with local authorities to prevent duplication.

7.28.A20. The minimum ceiling height shall be 7 feet 10 inches (2.39 meters), with the following exceptions:

a. Boiler rooms shall have ceiling clearances not less than 2 feet 6 inches (76.20 centimeters) above the main boiler header and connecting piping.

b. Ceilings in radiographic, operating and delivery rooms, and other rooms containing ceiling-mounted equipment or ceiling-mounted surgical light fixtures shall be of sufficient height to accommodate the equipment or fixtures and their normal movement.

c. Ceilings in corridors, storage rooms, and toilet rooms shall be not less than 7 feet 8 inches (2.34 meters) in height. Ceiling heights in small, normally unoccupied spaces may be reduced.

d. Suspended tracks, rails, and pipes located in the traffic path for patients in beds and/or on stretchers, including those in inpatient service areas, shall be not less than 7 feet (2.13 meters) above the floor. Clearances in other areas may be 6 feet 8 inches (2.03 meters).

e. Where existing structures make the above ceiling clearance impractical, clearances shall be as required to avoid injury to individuals up to 6 feet 4 inches (1.93 meters) tall.

f. Seclusion treatment rooms shall have a minimum ceiling height of 9 feet (2.74 meters).

7.28.A21. Recreation rooms, exercise rooms, equipment rooms, and similar spaces where impact noises may be generated shall not be located directly over patient bed areas or delivery and operating suites, unless special provisions are made to minimize such noise.

7.28.A22. Rooms containing heat-producing equipment, such as boiler or heater rooms or laundries, shall be insulated and ventilated to prevent the floor surface above and/or the adjacent walls of occupied areas from exceeding a temperature of 10°F (6°C) above ambient room temperature.

7.28.A23. The noise reduction criteria shown in Table 1 shall apply to partitions, floors, and ceiling construction in patient areas.

7.28.B. Finishes

7.28.B1. Cubicle curtains and draperies shall be noncombustible or flame-retardant, and shall pass both the large- and small-scale tests of NFPA 701 when applicable.

7.28.B2. Materials and certain plastics known to produce noxious gases when burned shall not be used for mattresses, upholstery, and other items insofar as practical. (Typical "hard" floor coverings such as vinyl, vinyl composition, and rubber normally do not create a major fire or smoke problem.)

7.28.B3. Floors in areas and rooms in which flammable anesthetic agents are stored or administered shall comply with NFPA 99. Conductive flooring may be omitted in anesthetizing areas where a written resolution is signed by the hospital board stating that no flammable anesthetic agents will be used and appropriate notices are permanently and conspicuously affixed to the wall in each such area and room.

7.28.B4. Floor materials shall be easily cleanable and appropriately wear-resistant for the location. Floors in areas used for food preparation or food assembly shall be water-resistant. Floor surfaces, including tile joints, shall be resistant to food acids. In all areas subject to frequent wet-cleaning methods, floor materials shall not be physically affected by germicidal cleaning solutions. Floors subject to traffic while wet (such as shower and bath areas, kitchens, and similar work areas) shall have a nonslip surface.

7.28.B5. In new construction or major renovation work, the floors and wall bases of all operating rooms and any delivery rooms used for caesarean sections shall be monolithic and joint free. The floors and wall bases of kitchens, soiled workrooms, and other areas subject to frequent wet cleaning shall also be homogenous, but may have tightly sealed joints.

7.28.B6. Wall finishes shall be washable. In the vicinity of plumbing fixtures, wall finishes shall be smooth and water-resistant.

In dietary and food preparation areas, wall construction, finish, and trim, including the joints between the walls and the floors, shall be free of insect- and rodent-harboring spaces.

In operating rooms, delivery rooms for caesarean sections, isolation rooms, and sterile processing rooms, wall finishes shall be free of fissures, open joints, or crevices that may retain or permit passage of dirt particles.

7.28.B7. Floors and walls penetrated by pipes, ducts, and conduits shall be tightly sealed to minimize entry of rodents and insects. Joints of structural elements shall be similarly sealed.

7.28.B8. Ceilings, including exposed structure in areas normally occupied by patients or staff in food-preparation and food-storage areas, shall be cleanable with routine housekeeping equipment. Acoustic and lay-in ceiling, where used, shall not interfere with infection control.

In dietary areas and in other areas where dust fallout may present a problem, provide suspended ceilings.

In operating rooms, delivery rooms for caesarean sections, isolation rooms, and sterile processing rooms, provide ceilings that contain a minimum number of fissures, open joints, or crevices and minimize retention or passage of dirt particles.

In psychiatric patient rooms, toilets, and seclusion rooms, ceiling construction shall be monolithic to inhibit possible escape or suicide. Ceiling-mounted air and lighting devices shall be security type. Ceiling-mounted fire prevention sprinkler heads shall be of the concealed type.

7.28.B9. Rooms used for protective isolation shall not have carpeted floors and shall have monolithic ceilings.

7.29 Design and Construction, Including Fire-Resistant Standards

7.29.A. Design
Every building and portion thereof shall be designed and constructed to sustain all live and dead loads, including seismic and other environmental forces, in accordance with accepted engineering practices and standards as prescribed by local jurisdiction or by one of the model building codes. (See Section 1.1.A.)

7.29.B. Construction
Construction shall comply with the applicable requirements of NFPA 101, the standards contained herein, and the requirements of authorities having jurisdiction. If there are no applicable local codes, one of the recognized model building codes shall be used (see Section 1.5).

Note: NFPA 101 generally covers fire/safety requirements only, whereas most model codes also apply to structural elements. The fire/safety items of NFPA 101 would take precedence over other codes in case of conflict. Appropriate application of each would minimize problems. For example, some model codes require closers on all patient doors. NFPA 101 recognizes the potential fire/safety problems of this requirement and stipulates that if closers are used for patient room doors, smoke detectors should also be provided within each affected patient room.

7.29.C. Freestanding Buildings
Separate freestanding buildings for the boiler plant, laundry, shops, general storage or other nonpatient contact areas shall be built in accordance with applicable building codes for such occupancy.

7.29.D. Interior Finishes
Interior finishing materials shall comply with the flame-spread limitations and the smoke-production limitations indicated in NFPA 101. This does not apply to minor quantities of wood or other trim (see NFPA 101) or to wall covering less than four mil thick applied over a non-combustible base.

7.29.E. Insulation Materials
Building insulation materials, unless sealed on all sides and edges with noncombustible material, shall have a flame-spread rating of 25 or less and a smoke-developed rating of 150 or less when tested in accordance with NFPA 255.

7.29.F. Provisions for Disasters (See also Section 1.4.)

7.29.F1. An emergency-radio communication system shall be provided in each facility. This system shall operate independently of the building's service and emergency power systems during emergencies. The system shall have frequency capabilities to communicate with state emergency communication networks. Additional communication capabilities will be required of facilities containing a formal community emergency-trauma service or other specialty services (such as regional pediatric critical care units) that utilize staffed patient transport units.

7.29.F2. Unless specifically approved, hospitals shall not be built in areas subject to damage or inaccessibility due to natural floods. Where facilities may be subject to wind or water hazards, provision shall be made to ensure continuous operation.

7.30 Special Systems

7.30.A. General

7.30.A1 Prior to acceptance of the facility, all special systems shall be tested and operated to demonstrate to the owner or his designated representative that the installation and performance of these systems conform to design intent. Test results shall be documented for maintenance files.

7.30.A2. Upon completion of the special systems equipment installation contract, the owner shall be furnished with a complete set of manufacturers' operating, maintenance, and preventive maintenance instructions, a parts lists, and complete procurement information including equipment numbers and descriptions. Operating staff persons shall also be provided with instructions for proper operation of systems and equipment. Required information shall include all safety or code ratings as needed.

7.30.A3. Insulation shall be provided surrounding special system equipment to conserve energy, protect personnel, and reduce noise.

7.30.B. Elevators
All hospitals having patient facilities (such as bedrooms, dining rooms, or recreation areas) or critical services (such as operating, delivery, diagnostic, or therapeutic) located on other than the grade-level entrance floor shall have electric or hydraulic elevators. Installation and testing of elevators shall comply with ANSI/ASME A17.1 for new construction and ANSI/ASME A17.3 for existing facilities. (See ASCE 7-93 for seismic design and control systems requirements for elevators.)

7.30.B1. In the absence of an engineered traffic study the following guidelines for number of elevators shall apply:

a. At least one hospital-type elevator shall be installed when 1 to 59 patient beds are located on any floor other than the main entrance floor.

b. At least two hospital-type elevators shall be installed when 60 to 200 patient beds are located on floors other than the main entrance floor, or where the major inpatient services are located on a floor other than those containing patient beds. (Elevator service may be reduced for those floors providing only partial inpatient services.)

c. At least three hospital-type elevators shall be installed where 201 to 350 patient beds are located on floors other than the main entrance floor, or where the major inpatient services are located on a floor other than those containing patient beds. (Elevator service may be reduced for those floors which provide only partial inpatient services.)

d. For hospitals with more than 350 beds, the number of elevators shall be determined from a study of the hospital plan and the expected vertical transportation requirements.

*7.30.B2. Hospital-type elevator cars shall have inside dimensions that accommodate a patient bed with attendants. Cars shall be at least 5 feet 8 inches (1.73 meters) wide by 9 feet (2.74 meters) deep. Car doors shall have a clear opening of not less than 4 feet (1.22 meters) wide and 7 feet (2.13 meters) high. In renovations, existing elevators that can accommodate patient beds used in the facility will not be required to be increased in size.

Note: Additional elevators installed for visitors and material handling may be smaller than noted above, within restrictions set by standards for disabled access.

7.30.B3. Elevators shall be equipped with a two-way automatic level-maintaining device with an accuracy of ± ¼ inch (± 0.64 centimeters).

7.30.B4. Each elevator, except those for material handling, shall be equipped with an independent keyed switch for staff use for bypassing all landing button calls and responding to car button calls only.

7.30.B5. Elevator call buttons and controls shall not be activated by heat or smoke. Light beams, if used for operating door reopening devices without touch, shall be used in combination with door-edge safety devices and shall be interconnected with a system of smoke detectors. This is so that the light control feature will be overridden or disengaged should it encounter smoke at any landing.

7.30.B6. Field inspections and tests shall be made and the owner shall be furnished with written certification stating that the installation meets the requirements set forth in this section as well as all applicable safety regulations and codes.

7.30.C. Waste Processing Services

7.30.C1. Storage and disposal. Facilities shall be provided for sanitary storage and treatment or disposal of waste using techniques acceptable to the appropriate health and environmental authorities. The functional program shall stipulate the categories and volumes of waste for disposal and shall stipulate the methods of disposal for each.

7.30.C2. Medical waste. Medical waste shall be disposed of either by incineration or other approved technologies. Incinerators or other major disposal equipment may be shared by two or more institutions.

a. Incinerators or other major disposal equipment may also be used to dispose of other medical waste where local regulations permit. Equipment shall be designed for the actual quantity and type of waste to be destroyed and should meet all applicable regulations.

b. Incinerators with fifty-pounds-per-hour or greater capacities shall be in a separate room or outdoors; those with lesser capacities may be located in a separate area within the facility boiler room. Rooms and areas containing incinerators shall have adequate space and facilities for incinerator charging and cleaning, as well as necessary clearances for work and maintenance. Provisions shall be made for operation, temporary storage, and disposal of materials so that odors and fumes do not drift back into occupied areas. Existing approved incinerator installations, which are not in separate rooms or outdoors, may remain unchanged provided they meet the above criteria.

c. The design and construction of incinerators and trash chutes shall comply with NFPA 82.

*d. See Appendix A. Heat recovery.

*e. See Appendix A. Environmental guidelines.

7.30.C3. Nuclear Waste Disposal. See *Code of Federal Regulations,* title X, parts 20 and 35, concerning the handling and disposal of nuclear materials in health care facilities.

7.31 Mechanical Standards

7.31.A. General

7.31.A1. The mechanical system should be designed for overall efficiency and appropriate life-cycle cost. Details for cost-effective implementation of design features are interrelated and too numerous (as well as too basic) to list individually. Recognized engineering procedures shall be followed for the most economical and effective results. A well-designed system can generally achieve energy efficiency at minimal additional cost and simultaneously provide improved patient comfort. Different geographic areas may have climatic and use conditions that favor one system over another in terms of overall cost and efficiency. In no case shall patient care or safety be sacrificed for conservation.

Mechanical, electrical, and HVAC equipment may be located either internally or externally, or in separate buildings.

7.31.A2. Remodeling and work in existing facilities may present special problems. As practicality and funding permit, existing insulation, weather stripping, etc., should be brought up to standard for maximum economy and efficiency. Consideration shall be given to additional work that may be needed to achieve this.

7.31.A3. Facility design consideration shall include site, building mass, orientation, configuration, fenestration, and other features relative to passive and active energy systems.

7.31.A4. Insofar as practical, the facility should include provisions for recovery of waste cooling and heating energy (ventilation, exhaust, water and steam discharge, cooling towers, incinerators, etc.).

7.31.A5. Facility design consideration shall include recognized energy-saving mechanisms such as variable-air-volume systems, load shedding, programmed controls for unoccupied periods (nights and weekends, etc.) and use of natural ventilation, site and climatic conditions permitting. Systems with excessive installation and/or maintenance costs that negate long-range energy savings should be avoided.

7.31.A6. Air-handling systems shall be designed with an economizer cycle where appropriate to use outside air. (Use of mechanically circulated outside air does not reduce need for filtration.)

It may be practical in many areas to reduce or shut down mechanical ventilation during appropriate climatic and patient-care conditions and to use open windows for ventilation.

7.31.A7. Mechanical equipment, ductwork, and piping shall be mounted on vibration isolators as required to prevent unacceptable structure-borne vibration.

7.31.A8. Supply and return mains and risers for cooling, heating, and steam systems shall be equipped with valves to isolate the various sections of each system. Each piece of equipment shall have valves at the supply and return ends.

7.31.B. Thermal and Acoustical Insulation

7.31.B1. Insulation within the building shall be provided to conserve energy, protect personnel, prevent vapor condensation, and reduce noise.

7.31.B2. Insulation on cold surfaces shall include an exterior vapor barrier. (Material that will not absorb or transmit moisture will not require a separate vapor barrier.)

7.31.B3. Insulation, including finishes and adhesives on the exterior surfaces of ducts, piping, and equipment, shall have a flame-spread rating of 25 or less and a smoke-developed rating of 50 or less as determined by an independent testing laboratory in accordance with NFPA 255.

7.31.B4. If duct lining is used, it shall be coated and sealed, and shall meet ASTM C1071. These linings (including coatings, adhesives, and exterior surface insulation on pipes and ducts in spaces used as air supply plenums) shall have a flame-spread rating of 25 or less and a smoke-developed rating of 50 or less, as determined by an independent testing laboratory in accordance with NFPA 255. If existing lined ductwork is reworked in a renovation project, the liner seams and punctures shall be resealed.

7.31.B5. Duct linings exposed to air movement shall not be used in ducts serving operating rooms, delivery rooms, LDR rooms, nurseries, protective environment rooms, and critical care units. This requirement shall not apply to mixing boxes and acoustical traps that have special coverings over such lining.

7.31.B6. Existing accessible insulation within areas of facilities to be modernized shall be inspected, repaired, and/or replaced, as appropriate.

7.31.B7. Duct lining shall not be installed within 15 feet (4.57 meters) downstream of humidifiers.

7.31.C. Steam and Hot Water Systems

7.31.C1. Boilers shall have the capacity, based upon the net ratings published by the Hydronics Institute or another acceptable national standard, to supply the normal heating, hot water, and steam requirements of all systems and equipment. Their number and arrangement shall accommodate facility needs despite the breakdown or routine maintenance of any one boiler. The capacity of the remaining boiler(s) shall be sufficient to provide hot water service for clinical, dietary, and patient use; steam for sterilization and dietary purposes; and heating for operating, delivery, birthing, labor, recovery, intensive care, nursery, and general patient rooms. However, reserve capacity for facility space heating is not required in geographic areas where a design dry-bulb temperature of 25°F (–4°C) or more represents not less than 99 percent of the total hours in any one heating month as noted in ASHRAE's *Handbook of Fundamentals,* under the "Table for Climatic Conditions for the United States."

7.31.C2. Boiler accessories including feed pumps, heat-circulating pumps, condensate return pumps, fuel oil pumps, and waste heat boilers shall be connected and installed to provide both normal and standby service.

7.31.D. Air Conditioning, Heating, and Ventilation Systems

7.31.D1. All rooms and areas in the facility used for patient care shall have provisions for ventilation. The ventilation rates shown in Table 2 shall be used only as minimum standards; they do not preclude the use of higher, more appropriate rates. Though natural window ventilation for nonsensitive areas and patient rooms may be employed, weather permitting, availability of mechanical ventilation should be considered for use in interior areas and during periods of temperature extremes. Fans serving exhaust systems shall be located at the discharge end and shall be readily serviceable. Air supply and exhaust in rooms for which no minimum total air change rate is noted may vary down to zero in response to room load. For rooms listed in Table 2, where VAV systems are used, minimum total air change shall be within limits noted. Temperature control shall also comply with these standards. To maintain asepsis control, airflow supply and exhaust should generally be controlled to ensure movement of air from "clean" to "less clean" areas, especially in critical areas. The ventilation systems shall be designed and balanced according to the requirements shown in Table 2 and in the applicable notes.

7.31.D2. Exhaust systems may be combined to enhance the efficiency of recovery devices required for energy conservation. Local exhaust systems shall be used whenever possible in place of dilution ventilation to reduce exposure to hazardous gases, vapors, fumes, or mists.

7.31.D3. Fresh air intakes shall be located at least 25 feet (7.62 meters) from exhaust outlets of ventilating systems, combustion equipment stacks, medical-surgical vacuum systems, plumbing vents, or areas that may collect vehicular exhaust or other noxious fumes. (Prevailing winds and/or proximity to other structures may require greater clearances.) Plumbing and vacuum vents that terminate at a level above the top of the air intake may be located as close as 10 feet (3.05 meters). The bottom of outdoor air intakes serving central systems shall be as high as practical, but at least 6 feet (1.83 meters) above ground level, or, if installed above the roof, 3 feet (91 centimeters) above roof level. Exhaust outlets from areas that may be contaminated shall be above roof level and arranged to minimize recirculation of exhaust air into the building.

7.31.D4. In new construction and major renovation work, air supply for operating and delivery rooms shall be from ceiling outlets near the center of the work area. Return air shall be near the floor level. Each operating and delivery room shall have at least two return-air inlets located as remotely from each other as practical. (Design

should consider turbulence and other factors of air movement to minimize fall of particulates onto sterile surfaces.) Where extraordinary procedures, such as organ transplants, justify special designs, installation shall properly meet performance needs as determined by applicable standards. These special designs should be reviewed on a case-by-case basis.

7.31.D5. Air supply for rooms used for invasive procedures shall be at or near the ceiling. Return or exhaust air inlets shall be near the floor level. Exhaust grills for anesthesia evacuation and other special applications shall be permitted to be installed in the ceiling.

*7.31.D6. Each space routinely used for administering inhalation anesthesia and inhalation analgesia shall be served by a scavenging system to vent waste gases. If a vacuum system is used, the gas-collecting system shall be arranged so that it does not disturb patients' respiratory systems. Gases from the scavenging system shall be exhausted directly to the outside. The anesthesia evacuation system may be combined with the room exhaust system, provided that the part used for anesthesia gas scavenging exhausts directly to the outside and is not part of the recirculation system. Scavenging systems are not required for areas where gases are used only occasionally, such as the emergency room, offices for routine dental work, etc. Acceptable concentrations of anesthetizing agents are unknown at this time. The absence of specific data makes it difficult to set specific standards. However, any scavenging system should be designed to remove as much of the gas as possible from the room environment. It is assumed that anesthetizing equipment will be selected and maintained to minimize leakage and contamination of room air.

7.31.D7. The bottoms of ventilation (supply/return) openings shall be at least 3 inches (7.62 centimeters) above the floor.

7.31.D8. All central ventilation or air conditioning systems shall be equipped with filters with efficiencies equal to, or greater than, those specified in Table 3. Where two filter beds are required, filter bed no. 1 shall be located upstream of the air conditioning equipment and filter bed no. 2 shall be downstream of any fan or blowers. Filter efficiencies, tested in accordance with ASHRAE 52-92, shall be average. Filter frames shall be durable and proportioned to provide an airtight fit with the enclosing ductwork. All joints between filter segments and enclosing ductwork shall have gaskets or seals to provide a positive seal against air leakage. A manometer shall be installed across each filter bed having a required efficiency of 75 percent or more including hoods requiring HEPA filters.

*7.31.D9. If duct humidifiers are located upstream of the final filters, they shall be located at least 15 feet (4.57 meters) upstream of the final filters. Ductwork with duct-mounted humidifiers shall have a means of water removal. An adjustable high-limit humidistat shall be located downstream of the humidifier to reduce the potential of condensation inside the duct. All duct take-offs should be sufficiently downstream of the humidifier to ensure complete moisture absorption. Steam humidifiers shall be used. Reservoir-type water spray or evaporative pan humidifiers shall not be used.

7.31.D10. Air-handling duct systems shall be designed with accessibility for duct cleaning, and shall meet the requirements of NFPA 90A.

7.31.D11. Ducts that penetrate construction intended to protect against X-ray, magnetic, RFI, or other radiation shall not impair the effectiveness of the protection.

7.31.D12. Fire and smoke dampers shall be constructed, located, and installed in accordance with the requirements of NFPA 101, 90A, and the specific damper's listing requirements. Fans, dampers, and detectors shall be interconnected so that damper activation will not damage ducts. Maintenance access shall be provided at all dampers. All damper locations should be shown on design drawings. Dampers should be activated by fire or smoke sensors, not by fan cutoff alone. Switching systems for restarting fans may be installed for fire department use in venting smoke after a fire has been controlled. However, provisions should be made to avoid possible damage to the system due to closed dampers. When smoke partitions are required, heating, ventilation, and air conditioning zones shall be coordinated with compartmentation insofar as practical to minimize need to penetrate fire and smoke partitions.

7.31.D13. Hoods and safety cabinets may be used for normal exhaust of a space provided that minimum air change rates are maintained. If air change standards in Table 2 do not provide sufficient air for proper operation of exhaust hoods and safety cabinets (when in use), supplementary makeup air (filtered and preheated) shall be provided around these units to maintain the required airflow direction and exhaust velocity. Use of makeup air will avoid dependence upon infiltration from outdoor and/or from contaminated areas. Makeup systems for hoods shall be arranged to minimize "short circuiting" of air and to avoid reduction in air velocity at the point of contaminant capture.

7.31.D14. Laboratory hoods shall meet the following general standards:

a. Have an average face velocity of at least 75 feet per minute (0.38 meters per second).

b. Be connected to an exhaust system to the outside which is separate from the building exhaust system.

c. Have an exhaust fan located at the discharge end of the system.

d. Have an exhaust duct system of noncombustible corrosion-resistant material as needed to meet the planned usage of the hood.

7.31.D15. Laboratory hoods shall meet the following special standards:

a. Fume hoods, and their associated equipment in the air stream, intended for use with perchloric acid and other strong oxidants, shall be constructed of stainless steel or other material consistent with special exposures, and be provided with a water wash and drain system to permit periodic flushing of duct and hood. Electrical equipment intended for installation within such ducts shall be designed and constructed to resist penetration by water. Lubricants and seals shall not contain organic materials. When perchloric acid or other strong oxidants are only transferred from one container to another, standard laboratory fume hoods and the associated equipment may be used in lieu of stainless steel construction.

b. In new construction and major renovation work, each hood used to process infectious or radioactive materials shall have a minimum face velocity of 90–110 feet per minute (0.45–0.56 meters per second) with suitable pressure-independent air modulating devices and alarms to alert staff of fan shutdown or loss of airflow. Each shall also have filters with a 99.97 percent efficiency (based on the dioctyl-phthalate [DOP] test method) in the exhaust stream, and be designed and equipped to permit the safe removal, disposal, and replacement of contaminated filters. Filters shall be as close to the hood as practical to minimize duct contamination. Fume hoods intended for use with radioactive isotopes shall be constructed of stainless steel or other material suitable for the particular exposure and shall comply with NFPA 801, Facilities for Handling Radioactive Materials. Note: Radioactive isotopes used for injections, etc., without probability of airborne particulates or gases may be processed in a clean-workbench-type hood where acceptable to the Nuclear Regulatory Commission.

7.31.D16. Exhaust hoods handling grease-laden vapors in food preparation centers shall comply with NFPA 96. All hoods over cooking ranges shall be equipped with grease filters, fire extinguishing systems, and heat-actuated fan controls. Cleanout openings shall be provided every 20 feet (6.10 meters) and at changes in direction in the horizontal exhaust duct systems serving these hoods. (Horizontal runs of ducts serving range hoods should be kept to a minimum.)

7.31.D17. The ventilation system for anesthesia storage rooms shall conform to the requirements of NFPA 99, including the gravity option. Mechanically operated air systems are optional in this room.

7.31.D18. The ventilation system for the space that houses ethylene oxide (ETO) sterilizers should be designed to:

a. Provide a dedicated (not connected to a return air or other exhaust system) exhaust system. Refer to 29 CFR Part 1910.1047.

b. All source areas shall be exhausted, including the sterilizer equipment room, service/aeration areas, over the sterilizer door, and the aerator. If the ETO cylinders are not located in a well-ventilated, unoccupied equipment space, an exhaust hood shall be provided over the cylinders. The relief valve shall be terminated in a well-ventilated, unoccupied equipment space, or outside the building. If the floor drain which the sterilizer(s) discharges to is not located in a well-ventilated, unoccupied equipment space, an exhaust drain cap shall be provided (coordinate with local codes).

c. Ensure that general airflow is away from sterilizer operator(s).

d. Provide a dedicated exhaust duct system for ETO. The exhaust outlet to the atmosphere should be at least 25 feet (7.62 meters) away from any air intake.

7.31.D19. An audible and visual alarm shall activate in the sterilizer work area, and a 24-hour staffed location, upon loss of airflow in the exhaust system.

7.31.D20. Rooms with fuel-fired equipment shall be provided with sufficient outdoor air to maintain equipment combustion rates and to limit workstation temperatures.

7.31.D21. Gravity exhaust may be used, where conditions permit, for nonpatient areas such as boiler rooms, central storage, etc.

7.31.D22. The energy-saving potential of variable air volume systems is recognized and these standards herein are intended to maximize appropriate use of that system. Any system utilized for occupied areas shall include provisions to avoid air stagnation in interior spaces where thermostat demands are met by temperatures of surrounding areas.

7.31.D23. Special consideration shall be given to the type of heating and cooling units, ventilation outlets, and appurtenances installed in patient-occupied areas of psychiatric units. The following shall apply:

a. All air grilles and diffusers shall be of a type that prohibits the insertion of foreign objects. All exposed fasteners shall be tamper-resistant.

b. All convector or HVAC enclosures exposed in the room shall be constructed with rounded corners and shall have enclosures fastened with tamper-resistant screws.

c. HVAC equipment shall be of a type that minimizes the need for maintenance within the room.

*7.31.D24. Rooms or booths used for sputum induction, aerosolized pentamadine treatments, and other high-risk cough-inducing procedures shall be provided with local exhaust ventilation. See Table 2 for ventilation requirements.

7.31.D25. Non-central air handling systems, i.e., individual room units that are used for heating and cooling purposes (fan-coil units, heat pump units, etc.), shall be equipped with permanent (cleanable) or replaceable filters. The filters shall have a minimum efficiency of 68 percent weight arrestance. These units may be used as recirculating units only. All outdoor air requirements shall be met by a separate central air handling system with the proper filtration, as noted in Table 3.

7.31.E. Plumbing and Other Piping Systems
Unless otherwise specified herein, all plumbing systems shall be designed and installed in accordance with *National Standard Plumbing Code.*

7.31.E1. The following standards shall apply to plumbing fixtures:

a. The material used for plumbing fixtures shall be non-absorptive and acid-resistant.

b. Water spouts used in lavatories and sinks shall have clearances adequate to avoid contaminating utensils and the contents of carafes, etc.

c. General handwashing facilities used by medical and nursing staff and all lavatories used by patients and food handlers shall be trimmed with valves that can be operated without hands. (Single lever or wrist blade devices may be used.) Blade handles used for this purpose shall not exceed 4½ inches (11.43 cm) in length. Handles on clinical sinks shall be at least 6 inches (15.24 cm) long. Freestanding scrub sinks and lavatories used for scrubbing in procedure rooms shall be trimmed with foot, knee, or ultrasonic controls (no single lever wrist blades).

d. Clinical sinks shall have an integral trap wherein the upper portion of the water trap provides a visible seal.

e. Showers and tubs shall have nonslip walking surfaces.

7.31.E2. The following standards shall apply to potable water supply systems:

a. Systems shall be designed to supply water at sufficient pressure to operate all fixtures and equipment during maximum demand. Supply capacity for hot- and cold-water piping shall be determined on the basis of fixture units, using recognized engineering standards. When the ratio of plumbing fixtures to occupants is proportionally more than required by the building occupancy and is in excess of 1,000 plumbing fixture units, a diversity factor is permitted.

b. Each water service main, branch main, riser, and branch to a group of fixtures shall have valves. Stop valves shall be provided for each fixture. Appropriate panels for access shall be provided at all valves where required.

c. Vacuum breakers shall be installed on hose bibbs and supply nozzles used for connection of hoses or tubing in laboratories, housekeeping sinks, bedpan-flushing attachments, and autopsy tables, etc.

d. Bedpan-flushing devices (may be cold water) shall be provided in each inpatient toilet room; however, installation is optional in psychiatric and alcohol-abuse units where patients are ambulatory.

e. Potable water storage vessels (hot and cold) not intended for constant use shall not be installed.

7.31.E3. The following standards shall apply to hot water systems:

a. The water-heating system shall have sufficient supply capacity at the temperatures and amounts indicated in Table 4. Water temperature is measured at the point of use or inlet to the equipment.

b. Hot-water distribution systems serving patient care areas shall be under constant recirculation to provide continuous hot water at each hot water outlet. The temperature of hot water for showers and bathing shall be appropriate for comfortable use but shall not exceed 110°F (43°C) (see Table 4).

7.31.E4. The following standards shall apply to drainage systems:

a. Drain lines from sinks used for acid waste disposal shall be made of acid-resistant material.

b. Drain lines serving some types of automatic blood-cell counters must be of carefully selected material that will eliminate potential for undesirable chemical reactions (and/or explosions) between sodium azide wastes and copper, lead, brass, and solder, etc.

c. Insofar as possible, drainage piping shall not be installed within the ceiling or exposed in operating and delivery rooms, nurseries, food preparation centers, food serving facilities, food storage areas, central services, electronic data processing areas, electric closets, and other sensitive areas. Where exposed overhead drain piping in these areas is unavoidable, special provisions shall be made to protect the space below from leakage, condensation, or dust particles.

d. Floor drains shall not be installed in operating and delivery rooms.

*e. If a floor drain is installed in cystoscopy, it shall contain a nonsplash, horizontal-flow flushing bowl beneath the drain plate.

f. Drain systems for autopsy tables shall be designed to positively avoid splatter or overflow onto floors or back siphonage and for easy cleaning and trap flushing.

g. Building sewers shall discharge into community sewerage. Where such a system is not available, the facility shall treat its sewage in accordance with local and state regulations.

h. Kitchen grease traps shall be located and arranged to permit easy access without the need to enter food preparation or storage areas. Grease traps shall be of capacity required and shall be accessible from outside of the building without need to interrupt any services.

i. Where plaster traps are used, provisions shall be made for appropriate access and cleaning.

j. In dietary areas, floor drains and/or floor sinks shall be of type that can be easily cleaned by removal of cover. Provide floor drains or floor sinks at all "wet" equipment (as ice machines) and as required for wet cleaning of floors. Provide removable stainless steel mesh in addition to grilled drain cover to prevent entry of large particles of waste which might cause stoppages. Location of floor drains and floor sinks shall be coordinated to avoid conditions where locations of equipment make removal of covers for cleaning difficult.

7.31.E5. The installation, testing, and certification of nonflammable medical gas and air systems shall comply with the requirements of NFPA 99. (See Table 5 for rooms that require station outlets.)

7.31.E6. Clinical vacuum system installations shall be in accordance with NFPA 99. (See Table 5 for rooms that require station outlets.)

7.31.E7. All piping, except control-line tubing, shall be identified. All valves shall be tagged, and a valve schedule shall be provided to the facility owner for permanent record and reference.

7.31.E8. When the functional program includes hemodialysis, continuously circulated filtered cold water shall be provided.

7.31.E9. Provide condensate drains for cooling coils of type that may be cleaned as needed without disassembly. (Unless specifically required by local authorities, traps are not required for condensate drains.) Provide air gap where condensate drains empty into floor drains. Provide heater elements for condensate lines in freezer or other areas where freezing may be a problem.

7.31.E10. No plumbing lines may be exposed overhead or on walls where possible accumulation of dust or soil may create a cleaning problem or where leaks would create a potential for food contamination.

7.32 Electrical Standards

7.32.A. General

7.32.A1. All electrical material and equipment, including conductors, controls, and signaling devices, shall be installed in compliance with applicable sections of NFPA 70 and NFPA 99 and shall be listed as complying with available standards of listing agencies, or other similar established standards where such standards are required.

7.32.A2. The electrical installations, including alarm, nurse call, and communication systems, shall be tested to demonstrate that equipment installation and operation is appropriate and functional. A written record of performance tests on special electrical systems and equipment shall show compliance with applicable codes and standards.

7.32.A3. Shielded isolation transformers, voltage regulators, filters, surge suppressors, and other safeguards shall be provided as required where power line disturbances are likely to affect data processing and/or automated laboratory or diagnostic equipment.

7.32.B. Services and Switchboards

Main switchboards shall be located in an area separate from plumbing and mechanical equipment and shall be accessible to authorized persons only. Switchboards shall be convenient for use, readily accessible for maintenance, away from traffic lanes, and located in dry, ventilated spaces free of corrosive or explosive fumes, gases, or any flammable material. Overload protective devices shall operate properly in ambient room temperatures.

7.32.C. Panelboards

Panelboards serving normal lighting and appliance circuits shall be located on the same floor as the circuits they serve. Panelboards serving critical branch emergency circuits shall be located on each floor that has major users (operating rooms, delivery suites, intensive care, etc.). Panelboards serving Life Safety emergency circuits may also serve floors above and/or below.

7.32.D. Lighting

7.32.D1. The Illuminating Engineering Society of North America (IES) has developed recommended lighting levels for health care facilities. The reader should refer to the *IES Handbook*.

7.32.D2. Approaches to buildings and parking lots, and all occupied spaces within buildings shall have fixtures that can be illuminated as necessary.

7.32.D3. Patient rooms shall have general lighting and night lighting. A reading light shall be provided for each patient. Reading light controls shall be readily accessible to the patient(s). Incandescent and halogen light sources which produce heat shall be avoided to prevent burns to the patient and/or bed linen. The light source should be covered by a diffuser or lens. Flexible light arms, if used, shall be mechanically controlled to prevent the lamp from contacting the bed linen. At least one night light fixture in each patient room shall be controlled at the room entrance. Lighting for coronary and intensive care bed areas shall permit staff observation of the patient while minimizing glare.

7.32.D4. Operating and delivery rooms shall have general lighting in addition to special lighting units provided at surgical and obstetrical tables. General lighting and special lighting shall be on separate circuits.

7.32.D5. Nursing unit corridors shall have general illumination with provisions for reducing light levels at night.

7.32.D6. Light intensity for staff and patient needs should generally comply with health care guidelines set forth in the IES publication. Consideration should be given to controlling intensity and/or wavelength to prevent harm to the patient's eyes (i.e., retina damage to premature infants and cataracts due to ultraviolet light).

Many procedures are available to satisfy lighting requirements, but the design should consider light quality as well as quantity for effectiveness and efficiency. While light levels in the IES publication are referenced herein, those publications include other useful guidance and recommendations that the designer is encouraged to follow.

7.32.D7. Consideration should be given to the special needs of the elderly. Excessive contrast in lighting levels that makes effective sight adaptation difficult should be minimized.

7.32.D8. A portable or fixed examination light shall be provided for examination, treatment, and trauma rooms.

7.32.D9. Light intensity of required emergency lighting shall generally comply with the IES recommendations. Egress and exit lighting shall comply with NFPA 101.

7.32.E. Receptacles

7.32.E1. Each operating and delivery room shall have at least six receptacles convenient to the head of the procedure table.

Each operating room shall have at least 16 simplex or eight duplex receptacles. Where mobile X-ray, laser, or other equipment requiring special electrical configurations is used, additional receptacles distinctively marked for X-ray or laser use shall be provided.

7.32.E2. Each patient room shall have duplex-grounded receptacles. There shall be one at each side of the head of each bed; one for television, if used; and one on every other wall. Receptacles may be omitted from exterior walls where construction or room configuration makes installation impractical. Nurseries shall have at least two duplex-grounded receptacles for each bassinet. Critical care areas as defined by NFPA 99 and NFPA 70, including pediatric and newborn intensive care units, shall have at least seven duplex outlets at the head of each bed, crib, or bassinet. Trauma and resuscitation rooms shall have eight duplex outlets located convenient to the head of each bed. Emergency department examination and treatment rooms shall have a minimum of six duplex outlets located convenient to the head of each bed. Approximately 50 percent of critical and emergency care outlets shall be connected to emergency system power and be so labelled. Each general care examination and treatment table and each work table shall have access to two duplex receptacles.

7.32.E3. Duplex-grounded receptacles for general use shall be installed approximately 50 feet (15.24 meters) apart in all corridors and within 25 feet (7.62 meters) of corridor ends. Receptacles in pediatric and psychiatric unit corridors shall be of the tamper resistant type. Special receptacles marked for X-ray use shall be installed in corridors of patient areas so that mobile equipment may be used anywhere within a patient room using a cord length of 50 feet (15.24 meters) or less. If the same mobile X-ray unit is used in operating rooms and in nursing areas, receptacles for X-ray use shall permit the use of one plug in all locations. *Where capacitive discharge or battery-powered X-ray units are used, special X-ray receptacles are not required.*

7.32.E4. Electrical receptacle cover plates or electrical receptacles supplied from the emergency systems shall be distinctively colored or marked for identification. If color is used for identification purposes, the same color shall be used throughout the facility.

7.32.E5. For renal dialysis units, two duplex receptacles shall be on each side of a patient bed or lounge chair. One duplex receptacle on each side of the bed shall be connected to emergency power.

7.32.F. Equipment

7.32.F1. At inhalation anesthetizing locations, all electrical equipment and devices, receptacles, and wiring shall comply with applicable sections of NFPA 99 and NFPA 70.

7.32.F2. Fixed and mobile X-ray equipment installations shall conform to articles 517 and 660 of NFPA 70.

7.32.F3. The X-ray film illuminator unit or units for displaying at least two films simultaneously shall be installed in each operating room, specified emergency treatment rooms, and X-ray viewing room of the radiology department. All illuminator units within one space or room shall have lighting of uniform intensity and color value.

7.32.F4. Ground-fault circuit interrupters (GFCI) shall comply with NFPA 70. *When ground-fault circuit interrupters are used in critical areas, provisions shall be made to ensure that other essential equipment is not affected by activation of one interrupter.*

7.32.F5. In areas such as critical care units and special nurseries where a patient may be treated with an internal probe or catheter connected to the heart, the ground system shall comply with applicable sections of NFPA 99 and NFPA 70.

7.32.F6. Special equipment is identified in the following sections: Critical Care Units, Newborn Nurseries, Pediatric and Adolescent Unit, Psychiatric Nursing Unit, Surgical Suites, Obstetrical Suite, Emergency Service, Imaging Suite, Nuclear Medicine, Laboratory Suite, Rehabilitation Therapy Department, Renal Dialysis Unit, Respiratory Therapy Service, Morgue, Pharmacy, Dietary Facilities, Administration and Public Areas, Medical Records, Central Services, General Stores, Linen Services.

These sections shall be consulted to ensure compatibility between programmatically defined equipment needs and appropriate power and other electrical connection needs.

7.32.F7. Special attention should be paid to safety hazards associated with equipment cabling. Every attempt should be made to minimize these hazards, where practical.

7.32.G. Nurses Calling System.

7.32.G1. In patient areas, each patient room shall be served by at least one calling station for two-way voice communication. Each bed shall be provided with a call device. Two call devices serving adjacent beds may be served by one calling station. Calls shall activate a visible signal in the corridor at the patient's door, in the clean workroom, in the soiled workroom, Medication, charting, clean linen storage, nourishment, equipment storage, and examination/treatment room(s) and at the nursing station of the nursing unit. In multi-corridor nursing units, additional visible signals shall be installed at corridor intersections. In rooms containing two or more calling stations, indicating lights shall be provided at each station. Nurses calling systems at each calling station shall be equipped with an indicating light which remains lighted as long as the voice circuit is operating.

7.32.G2. A nurses emergency call system shall be provided at each inpatient toilet, bath, sitz bath, and shower room. A nurses emergency call shall be accessible to a collapsed patient lying on the floor. Inclusion of a pull cord will satisfy this standard.

The emergency call shall be designed so that a signal activated at a patient's calling station will initiate a visible and audible signal distinct from the regular nurse calling system that can be turned off only at the patient calling station. The signal shall activate an annunciator panel at the nurse station, a visible signal in the corridor at the patient's door, and at other areas defined by the functional program. Provisions for emergency calls will also be needed in outpatient and treatment areas where patients may be subject to incapacitation.

7.32.G3. In areas such as critical care, recovery, and pre-op, where patients are under constant visual surveillance, the nurses call may be limited to a bedside button or station that activates a signal readily seen at the control station.

7.32.G4. A staff emergency assistance system for staff to summon additional assistance shall be provided in each operating, delivery, recovery, emergency examination and/or treatment area, and in critical care units, nurseries, special procedure rooms, cardiac catheterization rooms, stress-test areas, triage, outpatient surgery, admission and discharge areas, and areas for psychiatric patients including seclusion and security rooms, anterooms and toilet rooms serving them, communal toilet and bathing facility rooms, and dining, activity, therapy, exam, and treatment rooms. This system shall annunciate visually and audibly in the clean work room, in the soiled work room, medication, charting, clean linen storage, nourishment, equipment storage, and examination/treatment room(s) if provided and at the nursing station of the nursing unit with back up to another staffed area from which assistance can be summoned.

7.32.G5. In critical care units, recovery and pre-op, the call system shall include provisions for an emergency code resuscitation alarm to summon assistance from outside the unit.

7.32.G6. A nurse call is not required in psychiatric nursing units, but if it is included, provisions shall be made for easy removal, or for covering call button outlets. In psychiatric nursing units all hardware shall have tamper-resistant fasteners.

7.32.G7. Patient toilet rooms within Imaging Suite shall be equipped with a nurses emergency call.

7.32.G8. Toilet rooms in renal dialysis units shall be served by an emergency call. Call shall activate a signal at the nurses' station.

7.32.G9. Alternate technologies can be considered for emergency or nurse call systems. If radio frequency systems are utilized, consideration should be given to electromagnetic compatibility between internal and external sources.

7.32.H. Emergency Electric Service
Emergency power shall be provided for in accordance with NFPA 99, NFPA 101, and NFPA 110.

7.32.I. Fire Alarm
All health care occupancies shall be provided with a fire alarm system in accordance with NFPA 101 and NFPA 72.

7.32.J. Telecommunications and Information Systems

7.32.J1. Locations for terminating telecommunications and information system devices shall be provided.

7.32.J2. A room shall be provided for central equipment locations. Special air conditioning and voltage regulation shall be provided when recommended by the manufacturer.

Table 1

Sound Transmission Limitations
in General Hospitals

	Airborne sound transmission class (STC)[a]	
	Partitions	Floors
New construction		
Patient room to patient room	45	40
Public space to patient room[b]	55	40
Service areas to patient room[c]	65	45
Patient room access corridor[d]	45	45
Existing construction		
Patient room to patient room	35	40
Public space to patient room[b]	40	40
Service areas to patient room[c]	45	45

[a] Sound transmission class (STC) shall be determined by tests in accordance with methods set forth in ASTM E90 and ASTM E413. *Where partitions do not extend to the structure above, sound transmission through ceilings and composite STC performance must be considered.*

[b] Public space includes corridors (except patient room access corridors), lobbies, dining rooms, recreation rooms, treatment rooms, and similar space.

[c] Service areas include kitchens, elevators, elevator machine rooms, laundries, garages, maintenance rooms, boiler and mechanical equipment rooms, and similar spaces of high noise. Mechanical equipment located on the same floor or above patient rooms, offices, nurses stations, and similar occupied space shall be effectively isolated from the floor.

[d] Patient room access corridors contain composite walls with doors/windows and have direct access to patient rooms.

Table 2

Ventilation Requirements for Areas Affecting Patient Care in Hospitals and Outpatient Facilities[1]

Area designation	Air movement relationship to adjacent area[2]	Minimum air changes of outdoor air per hour[3]	Minimum total air changes per hour[4]	All air exhausted directly to outdoors[5]	Recirculated by means of room units[6]	Relative humidity[7] (%)	Design temperature[8] (degrees F/C)
SURGERY AND CRITICAL CARE							
Operating/surgical cystoscopic rooms[9]	Out	3	15	—	No	30-60	68–73 (20–23)
Delivery room[9]	Out	3	15	—	No	30-60	68–73 (20–23)
Recovery room[9]	—	2	6	—	No	30-60	70 (21)
Critical and intensive care	—	2	6	—	No	30-60	70-75 (21–24)
Treatment room[10]	—	—	6	—	—	—	75 (24)
Trauma room[10]	Out	3	15	—	No	45-60	70-75 (21–24)
Anesthesia gas storage	—	—	8	Yes	—	—	—
Endoscopy	—	2	6	—	No	30–60	68–73 (20–23)
Bronchoscopy	In	2	12	Yes	No	30–60	68–73 (20–23)
NURSING							
Patient room	—	2	2	—	—	—	70-75 (21–24)
Toilet room	In	—	10	Yes	—	—	—
Newborn nursery suite	—	2	6	—	No	30-60	75 (24)
Protective Environment Room[11]	Out	2	12	—	No	—	75 (24)
Airborne infection isolation room[12]	In	2	12	—	No	—	75 (24)
Isolation alcove or anteroom[11, 12]	In/Out	—	10	Yes	No	—	—
Labor/delivery/recovery	—	2	2	—	—	—	70-75 (21–24)
Labor/delivery/recovery/postpartum	—	2	2	—	—	—	70-75 (21–24)
Patient corridor	—	—	2	—	—	—	—
ANCILLARY							
Radiology[13]							
X-ray (surgical/critical care and catheterization)	Out	3	15	—	No	30-60	70-75 (21–24)
X-ray (diagnostic & treat.)	—	—	6	—	—	—	75 (24)
Darkroom	In	—	10	Yes	No	—	—
Laboratory							
General[14]	—	—	6	—	—	—	75 (24)
Biochemistry[14]	Out	—	6	—	No	—	75 (24)
Cytology	In	—	6	Yes	No	—	75 (24)
Glass washing	In	—	10	Yes	—	—	—
Histology	In	—	6	Yes	No	—	75 (24)
Microbiology[13]	In	—	6	Yes	No	—	75 (24)

Notes

[1] The ventilation rates in this table cover ventilation for comfort, as well as for asepsis and odor control in areas of acute care hospitals that directly affect patient care and are determined based on healthcare facilities being predominantly "No Smoking" facilities. Where smoking may be allowed, ventilation rates will need adjustment. Areas where specific ventilation rates are not given in the table shall be ventilated in accordance with ASHRAE Standard 62-1989, *Ventilation for Acceptable Indoor Air Quality,* and ASHRAE *Handbook of Applications*. Specialized patient care areas, including organ transplant units, burn units, specialty procedure rooms, etc., shall have additional ventilation provisions for air quality control as may be appropriate. OSHA standards and/or NIOSH criteria require special ventilation requirements for employee health and safety within health care facilities.

[2] Design of the ventilation system shall provide air movement which is generally from clean to less clean areas. If any form of variable air volume or load shedding system is used for energy conservation, it must not compromise the corridor-to-room pressure balancing relationships or the minimum air changes required by the table. Except where specifically permitted by exit corridor plenum provisions of NFPA 90A, the volume of infiltration and exfiltration shall not exceed 15 percent of the minimum total air changes per hour, or 50 cfm, whichever is larger, as defined by the table.

[3] To satisfy exhaust needs, replacement air from the outside is necessary. Table 2 does not attempt to describe specific amounts of outside air to be supplied to individual spaces except for certain areas such as those listed. Distribution of the outside air, added to the system to balance required exhaust, shall be as required by good engineering practice. Minimum outside air quantities shall remain constant while the system is in operation.

[4] Number of air changes may be reduced when the room is unoccupied if provisions are made to ensure that the number of air changes indicated is reestablished any time the space is being utilized. Adjustments shall include provisions so that the direction of air movement shall remain the same when the number of air changes is reduced. Areas not indicated as having continuous directional control may have ventilation systems shut down when space is unoccupied and ventilation is not otherwise needed, if the maximum infiltration or exfiltration permitted in Note 2 is not exceeded and if adjacent pressure balancing relationships are not compromised.

Table 2 *(continued)*

Ventilation Requirements for Areas Affecting Patient Care in Hospitals and Outpatient Facilities[1]

Area designation	Air movement relationship to adjacent area[2]	Minimum air changes of outdoor air per hour[3]	Minimum total air changes per hour[4]	All air exhausted directly to outdoors[5]	Recirculated by means of room units[6]	Relative humidity[7] (%)	Design temperature[8] (degrees F/C)
Laboratory *(continued)*							
Nuclear medicine	In	—	6	Yes	No	—	75 (24)
Pathology	In	—	6	Yes	No	—	75 (24)
Serology	Out	—	6	—	No	—	75 (24)
Sterilizing	In	—	10	Yes	—	—	—
Autopsy room	In	—	12	Yes	No	—	—
Nonrefrigerated body-holding room	In	—	10	Yes	—	—	70 (21)
Pharmacy	—	—	4	—	—	—	—
DIAGNOSTIC AND TREATMENT							
Examination room	—	—	6	—	—	—	75 (24)
Medication room	—	—	4	—	—	—	—
Treatment room	—	—	6	—	—	—	75 (24)
Physical therapy and hydrotherapy	In	—	6	—	—	—	75 (24)
Soiled workroom or soiled holding	In	—	10	Yes	No	—	—
Clean workroom or clean holding	—	—	4	—	—	—	—
STERILIZING AND SUPPLY							
ETO-sterilizer room	In	—	10	Yes	No	30–60	75 (24)
Sterilizer equipment room	In	—	10	Yes	—	—	—
Central medical and surgical supply							
Soiled or decontamination room	In	—	6	Yes	No	—	68–73 (20–23)
Clean workroom	Out	—	4	—	No	30–60	75 (24)
Sterile Storage	—	—	4	—	—	(Max) 70	—
SERVICE							
Food preparation center[14]	—	—	10	—	No	—	—
Warewashing	In	—	10	Yes	No	—	—
Dietary day storage	In	—	2	—	—	—	—
Laundry, general	—	—	10	Yes	—	—	—
Soiled linen (sorting and storage)	In	—	10	Yes	No	—	—
Clean linen storage	—	—	2	—	—	—	—
Soiled linen and trash chute room	In	—	10	Yes	No	—	—
Bedpan room	In	—	10	Yes	—	—	—
Bathroom	—	—	10	—	—	—	75 (24)
Janitor's closet	In	—	10	Yes	No	—	—

5 Air from areas with contamination and/or odor problems shall be exhausted to the outside and not recirculated to other areas. Note that individual circumstances may require special consideration for air exhaust to the outside, e.g., in intensive care units in which patients with pulmonary infection are treated, and rooms for burn patients.

*6 Recirculating room HVAC units refers to those local units that are used primarily for heating and cooling of air, and not disinfection of air. Because of cleaning difficulty and potential for buildup of contamination, recirculating room units shall not be used in areas marked "No." However, for airborne infection control, air may be recirculated within individual isolation rooms if HEPA filters are used. Isolation and intensive care unit rooms may be ventilated by reheat induction units in which only the primary air supplied from a central system passes through the reheat unit. Gravity-type heating or cooling units such as radiators or convectors shall not be used in operating rooms and other special care areas. See Appendix A for a description of recirculation units to be used in isolation rooms.

7 The ranges listed are the minimum and maximum limits where control is specifically needed.

8 Where temperature ranges are indicated, the systems shall be capable of maintaining the rooms at any point within the range. A single figure indicates a heating or cooling capacity of at least the indicated temperature. This is usually applicable when patients may be undressed and require a warmer environment. Nothing in these guidelines shall be construed as precluding the use of temperatures lower than those noted when the patients' comfort and medical conditions make lower temperatures desirable. Unoccupied areas such as storage rooms shall have temperatures appropriate for the function intended.

9 National Institute for Occupational Safety and Health (NIOSH) Criteria Documents regarding Occupational Exposure to Waste Anesthetic Gases and Vapors, and Control of Occupational Exposure to Nitrous Oxide indicate a need for both local exhaust (scavenging) systems and general ventilation of the areas in which the respective gases are utilized.

10 The term trauma room as used here is the operating room space in the emergency department or other trauma reception area that is used for emergency surgery. The first aid room and/or "emergency room" used for initial treatment of accident victims may be

(continued on next page)

ventilated as noted for the "treatment room." Treatment rooms used for Bronchoscopy shall be treated as Bronchoscopy rooms. Treatment rooms used for cryosurgery procedures with nitrous oxide shall contain provisions for exhausting waste gases.

*11 The protective environment airflow design specifications protect the patient from common environmental airborne infectious microbes (i.e., Aspergillus spores). These special ventilation areas shall be designed to provide directed airflow from the cleanest patient care area to less clean areas. These rooms shall be protected with HEPA filters at 99.97 percent efficiency for a 0.3 μm sized particle in the supply airstream. These interrupting filters protect patient rooms from maintenance-derived release of environmental microbes from the ventilation system components. Recirculation HEPA filters can be used to increase the equivalent room air exchanges. Constant volume airflow is required for consistent ventilation for the protected environment. If the facility determines that airborne infection isolation is necessary for protective environment patients, an anteroom should be provided. Rooms with reversible airflow provisions for the purpose of switching between protective environment and airborne infection isolation functions are not acceptable.

12 The infectious disease isolation room described in these guidelines is to be used for isolating the airborne spread of infectious diseases, such as measles, varicella, or tuberculosis. The design of airborne infection isolation (AII) rooms should include the provision for normal patient care during periods not requiring isolation precautions. Supplemental recirculating devices may be used in the patient room, to increase the equivalent room air exchanges; however, such recirculating devices do not provide the outside air requirements. Air may be recirculated within individual isolation rooms if HEPA filters are used. Rooms with reversible airflow provisions for the purpose of switching between protective environment and AII functions are not acceptable.

13 When required, appropriate hoods and exhaust devices for the removal of noxious gases or chemical vapors shall be provided (see Section 7.31.D1.n and o and NFPA 99).

14 Food preparation centers shall have ventilation systems whose air supply mechanisms are interfaced appropriately with exhaust hood controls or relief vents so that exfiltration or infiltration to or from exit corridors does not compromise the exit corridor restrictions of NFPA 90A, the pressure requirements of NFPA 96, or the maximum defined in the table. The number of air changes may be reduced or varied to any extent required for odor control when the space is not in use. See Section 7.31.D1.p.

Table 3

Filter Efficiencies for Central Ventilation and Air Conditioning Systems in General Hospitals

Area designation	No. filter beds	Filter bed no. 1 (%)	Filter bed no. 2 (%)
All areas for inpatient care, treatment, and diagnosis, and those areas providing direct service or clean supplies such as sterile and clean processing, etc.	2	30	90
Protective environment room	2	30	99.97
Laboratories	1	80	—
Administrative, bulk storage, soiled holding areas, food preparation areas, and laundries	1	30	—

Notes: Additional roughing or prefilters should be considered to reduce maintenance required for filters with efficiency higher than 75 percent. The filtration efficiency ratings are based on dust spot efficiency per ASHRAE 52-76.

Table 4

Hot Water Use—General Hospital

	Clinical	Dietary[†]	Laundry
Liters per second per bed*	.0033	.0020	.0021
Gallons per hour per bed*	3	2	2
Temperature (°C)**	43	49	71**
Temperature (°F)**	110	120	160**

† Provisions shall be made to provide 180°F (82°C) rinse water at warewasher. (May be by separate booster.)

* Quantities indicated for design demand of hot water are for general reference minimums and shall not substitute for accepted engineering design procedures using actual number and types of fixtures to be installed. Design will also be affected by temperatures of cold water used for mixing, length of run and insulation relative to heat loss, etc. As an example, total quantity of hot water needed will be less when temperature available at the outlet is very nearly that of the source tank and the cold water used for tempering is relatively warm.

**Provisions shall be made to provide 160°F (71°C) hot water at the laundry equipment when needed. (This may be by steam jet or separate booster heater.) However, it is emphasized that this does not imply that all water used would be at this temperature. Water temperatures required for acceptable laundry results will vary according to type of cycle, time of operation, and formula of soap and bleach as well as type and degree of soil. Lower temperatures may be adequate for most procedures in many facilities but the higher 160°F (71°C) should be available when needed for special conditions.

Table 5
Station Outlets for Oxygen, Vacuum (Suction), and Medical Air Systems

Section	Location	Oxygen	Vacuum	Medical Air
7.2.A	Patient Rooms (Medical and Surgical)	1 (one outlet accessible to each bed)	1 (one outlet) accessible to each bed)	—
7.2.B10	Examination/Treatment (Medical, Surgical, and Postpartum Care)	1	1	—
7.2.C/7.2.D	Isolation (Infectious and Protective) (Medical and Surgical)	1	1	—
7.2.E	Security Room (Medical, Surgical, and Postpartum)	1	1	—
7.3.A	Critical Care (General)	2	3	1
7.3.A14	Isolation (Critical)	2	3	1
7.3.B	Coronary Critical Care	2	2	1
7.3.D	Pediatric Critical Care	2	3	1
7.3.E	Newborn Intensive Care	3	3	3
7.4.B	Newborn Nursery (full-term)	1	1	1
7.5.A	Pediatric and Adolescent	1	1	1
7.5.B	Pediatric Nursery	1	1	1
7.6.A	Psychiatric Patient Rooms	—	—	—
7.6.D	Seclusion Treatment Room	—	—	—
7.7.A1	General Operating Room	2	3	
7.7.A2	Cardio, Ortho, Neurological	2	3	
7.7.A3	Orthopedic Surgery	2	3	
7.7.A4	Surgical Cysto and Endo	1	3	
7.7.B2	Post-Anesthetic Care Unit	1	3	
7.7.C9	Anesthesia Workroom	1 per workstation	—	1 per workstation
7.7.C14	Outpatient Recovery	1	3	
7.8.B2	Postpartum Bedroom	1	1	—
7.8.A3	Caesarean/Delivery Room	2	3	
7.8.A3(d)	Labor Room	1	1	
7.8.A3(e)	Recovery Room	1	3	
7.8.A4	Labor/Delivery/Recovery (LDR)	2	2	
7.8.A4	Labor/Delivery/Recovery/Postpartum (LDRP)	2	2	
7.9.C2	Initial Emergency Management per bed	1	1	
7.9.D3	Triage Area (Definitive Emergency Care)	1	1	—
7.9.D7	Definitive Emergency Care Exam/Treatment Rooms	1	1	1
7.9.D7	Definitive Emergency Care Holding Area	1	1	—
7.9.D8	Trauma/Cardiac Room(s)	2	3	1
7.9.D9	Orthopedic and Cast Room	1	1	
7.10.H	Cardiac Catheterization Lab	1	2	2
7.16.A2	Autopsy Room	—	1 per workstation	1 per workstation

8. NURSING FACILITIES

8.1 General Conditions

8.1.A. Applicability
This section covers the continuum of nursing services listed below, which may be provided within freestanding facilities or as distinct parts of a general hospital or other health care facility, and represents minimum requirements for new construction and shall not be applied to existing facilities unless major construction renovations (see Section 1.2.A) are undertaken.

The continuum of nursing services and facilities may be distinguished by the levels of care, staffing support areas and service areas provided and classified as:

> Nursing and skilled nursing facilities
> Special care facilities, including:
> > Subacute care facilities 8.7
> > Alzheimer's and other dementia units 8.8

Note: Specific requirements for each of the above special care facility types are addressed in the paragraphs noted above. For basic requirements see chapters 1 through 6. For requirements regarding swing beds see Section 7.1.E.

8.1.B. Ancillary Services
When the nursing facility is part of, or contractually linked with, another facility, services such as dietary, storage, pharmacy, linen services, and laundry may be shared insofar as practical. In some cases, all ancillary service requirements will be met by the principal facility and the only modifications necessary will be within the nursing facility. In other cases, programmatic concerns and requirements may dictate separate services.

8.1.C. Hospital Conversions
While there are similarities in the spatial arrangement of hospitals and nursing facilities, the service requirements of long-term care residents will require additional special design considerations. When a section of an acute-care facility is converted, it may be necessary to reduce the number of beds to provide space for long-term care services. Design shall maximize opportunities for ambulation and self-care, socialization, and independence and minimize the negative aspects of an institutional environment.

8.1.D. Site
See Sections 3.1 and 3.3 for requirements regarding location and environmental pollution control.

8.1.E. Roads
Roads shall be provided within the property for access to the main entrance and service areas. Fire department access shall be provided in accordance with local requirements. The property or campus shall be marked to identify emergency services or departments.

8.1.F. Parking
In the absence of local requirements, each nursing facility shall have parking space to satisfy the needs of residents, employees, staff, and visitors. The facility shall provide a minimum of one space for every four beds.

8.1.G. Program of Functions
The sponsor for each project shall provide a functional program for the facility (see Section 1.1.F of this document).

8.1.H. Services
Each nursing facility shall, as a minimum, contain the elements described within the applicable paragraphs of this section. However, when a project calls for the sharing or purchase of services, appropriate modifications or deletions in space and parking requirements may be made.

8.1.I. Renovation
See Section 1.2.

8.1.J. Provisions for Disasters
See Section 1.4.

8.1.K. Codes and Standards
See Section 1.5.

8.1.L. Energy Conservation
See Chapter 2.

8.1.M. Equipment
See Chapter 4.

8.1.N. Construction
See Chapter 5.

8.1.O. Record Drawings and Manuals
See Chapter 6.

8.2 Resident Unit

Each resident unit shall comply with the following:

*8.2.A. Size and Configuration
Resident units are groups of resident rooms, staff work areas, service areas and resident support areas, whose size and configuration are based upon organizational patterns of staffing, functional operations and communications, as provided in the functional program for the facility. In the absence of local requirements, consideration shall be given to restricting the size of the resident unit to 60 beds or a maximum travel distance from the staff station to a resident room door of 150 feet (45.72

meters). Arranging groups of resident rooms adjacent to decentralized service areas, optional satellite staff work areas, and optional decentralized resident support areas is acceptable.

8.2.B. Resident Rooms

Each resident room shall meet the following requirements:

8.2.B1. Maximum room occupancy in renovations (less than 50 percent change) shall be four residents; two residents in new construction.

8.2.B2. Room size (area and dimensions) shall be determined by analyzing the needs of the resident(s) to move about the room in a wheelchair, gain access to at least one side of his or her bed, turn and wheel around the bed, to gain access to a window and to the resident's toilet room, wardrobe locker, or closet, and to the resident's possessions or equipment, including chair, dresser, and night stand. Room size and configuration shall permit resident(s) options for bed location(s), make provision for visual privacy, and shall not be less than 120 square feet (11.15 square meters) in single-bed rooms and 100 square feet (9.29 square meters)per bed in multiple-bed rooms (exclusive of toilets, closets, lockers, wardrobes, alcoves or vestibules, in both cases). In renovations, minimum room areas (exclusive of toilets, closets, lockers, wardrobes, alcoves, or vestibules) shall be 100 square feet (9.29 square meters) in single-bed rooms and 80 square feet (7.43 square meters) per bed in multiple-bed rooms. In multiple-bed rooms, clearance shall allow for the movement of beds and equipment without disturbing residents.

8.2.B3. Each room shall have a window that meets the requirements of Section 8.15.A4.

8.2.B4. Handwashing facilities shall be provided in each resident room. They may be omitted from single-bed or two-bed rooms when such is located in an adjoining toilet room serving that room only.

8.2.B5. Each resident shall have access to a toilet room without having to enter the corridor area. One toilet room shall serve no more than two residents in new construction and no more than four beds or two resident rooms in renovation projects. The toilet room shall contain a water closet and handwashing facilities and (where permitted) a horizontal surface for the personal effects of each resident. The handwashing facilities may be omitted from a toilet room if each resident room served by that toilet contains handwashing facilities. Doors to toilet rooms may be hinged or, where local requirements permit, sliding or folding doors may be used, provided adequate provisions are made for acoustic privacy and resident safety.

8.2.B6. Each resident bedroom shall have a wardrobe, locker, or closet with minimum clear dimensions of 1 foot 10 inches (55.88 centimeters) depth by 1 foot 8 inches (50.80 centimeters); with a shelf and clothes rod to permit a vertically clear hanging space of 5 feet (1.52 meters) for full-length garments. (The shelf may be omitted if the unit provides at least two drawers and capacity for storing extra blankets, pillows, etc.)

8.2.B7. Visual privacy shall be provided for each resident in multiple-bed rooms. Design for privacy shall not restrict resident access to the toilet, handwashing facilities, or room entrance.

8.2.B8. Beds shall be no more than two deep from windows in new construction and three deep from windows in renovated construction.

8.2.B9. Provision should be made for wheelchairs within the room.

8.2.B10. The need for and number of required airborne infection isolation room(s) in nursing facilities shall be determined by an infection control risk assessment. When required, the airborne infection isolation room(s) shall comply with the general requirements of Section 7.2.C.

8.2.C. Service Areas

The size and features of each service area will depend upon the number and types of residents served. Although identifiable spaces are required for each indicated function, consideration will be given to multiple-use design solutions that provide equal, though unspecified, areas. Service areas may be arranged and located to serve more than one resident unit, but at least one such service area shall be provided on each resident floor unless noted otherwise. Except where the words room or office are used, service may be provided in a multipurpose area. The following service areas shall be located in or be readily accessible to each resident unit:

*8.2.C1. Staff work area(s). Resident units shall have staff work areas in central or decentralized direct care locations. Where caregiving is organized on a central staffing model, such work areas shall have space for charting, storage, and administrative activities. Where caregiving is decentralized, supervisory work areas need not accommodate charting activities, nor have direct visualization of resident rooms, because such functions shall be accomplished at the decentralized direct care staff work areas, which shall have space for charting and any storage or administrative functions required by the functional program. Depending upon the type of service and care plan to be provided, direct care staff work areas need not be encumbered with all of the provisions for a supervisory administrative staff work area. In some decentralized arrangements, caregiving functions may be accommodated at a piece of residential furniture (such as a table or a desk) or at a work counter recessed into an alcove off a corridor or activity space, with or without computer and communications equipment, storage facilities, etc.

8.2.C2. Toilet room(s). They shall contain water closets with handwashing facilities for staff and may be unisex.

8.2.C3. Lockable closets, drawers, or compartments shall be provided for safekeeping of staff personal effects such as handbags, etc.

8.2.C4. Staff lounge area(s). These areas shall be provided and may be shared by more than one resident unit or service.

8.2.C5. Clean utility room(s). This shall contain a counter and handwashing facilities and be sized to store clean and sterile supplies, as required by the functional program.

8.2.C6. Soiled utility or soiled holding room. This shall contain a clinical sink or equivalent flushing-rim fixture with a rinsing hose or a bed pan sanitizer, handwashing facilities, soiled linen receptacles, and waste receptacles in number and type as required by the functional program.

8.2.C7. Medication station. Provision shall be made for 24-hour distribution of medications. A medicine preparation room, a self-contained medicine dispensing unit, or other system may be used for this purpose. The medicine preparation room, if used, shall be visually controlled from the staff work area. It shall contain a work counter, sink, refrigerator, and locked storage for controlled drugs. It shall have a minimum area of 50 square feet (4.65 square meters). A self-contained medicine dispensing unit, if used, may be located at the staff work area, in the clean workroom, in an alcove, or in other space convenient for staff control. (Standard "cup" sinks provided in many self-contained units are not adequate for handwashing.)

8.2.C8. Clean linen storage. A separate closet or designated area shall be provided. If a closed-cart system is used, storage may be in an alcove where staff control can be exercised.

8.2.C9. Nourishment station. The area shall contain a work counter, refrigerator, storage cabinets, and a sink for serving nourishments between meals. Ice for residents' consumption shall be provided by ice-maker units. Ice-makers shall be located, designed, and installed to minimize noise (and may serve more than one nourishment station). The nourishment station shall include space for trays and dishes used for nonscheduled meal service and may also be used as a pantry for food service adjacent to a resident's dining room or area. Handwashing facilities shall be in or immediately accessible from the nourishment station.

8.2.C10. Storage. Space for wheelchairs and other equipment shall be located away from normal traffic.

8.2.C11. Resident bathing facilities. A minimum of one bathtub or shower shall be provided for every 20 residents (or a major fraction thereof) not otherwise served by bathing facilities in resident rooms. Residents shall have access to at least one bathtub room per floor or unit, sized to permit assisted bathing in a tub or shower. The bathtub in this room shall be accessible to residents in wheelchairs and the shower shall accommodate a shower gurney with fittings for a resident in a recumbent position. Other showers or tubs shall be in an individual room(s) or enclosure(s) with space for private use of the bathing fixture, for drying and dressing and access to a grooming location containing a sink, mirror, and counter or shelf.

A separate toilet shall be provided within or directly accessible to each resident's bathing facility without requiring entry into the general corridor. This may also serve as the toilet training facility.

8.3 Resident Support Areas

*8.3.A. Area Need
The space needed for dining and recreation shall be determined by considering (a) needs of residents to use adaptive equipment and mobility aids and receive assistance from support and service staff; and (b) the extent to which support programs shall be centralized or decentralized, as required by the functional program.

In new construction, the total area set aside for dining, resident lounges, and recreation areas shall be at least 35 square feet (3.25 square meters) per bed with a minimum total area of at least 225 square feet (20.92 square meters). At least 20 square feet (1.86 square meters) per bed shall be available for dining. Additional space may be required for outpatient day care programs.

For renovations, at least 14 square feet (1.30 square meters) per bed shall be available for dining. Additional space may be required for outpatient day care programs.

Nothing in these guidelines is intended to restrict a facility from providing additional square footage per resident beyond what is required herein for dining rooms, activity areas, and similar spaces.

8.3.B. Storage
Storage space(s) for supplies, resident needs, and recreation shall be provided near their points of use, as required by the functional program.

*8.4 Activities

If included in the functional program, the minimum requirements for new construction shall include:

8.4.A.
Storage for large items used for large group activities, e.g., recreation and exercise equipment, materials, supplies for religious services, etc., placed near the location of the planned activity and at the point of first use.

8.4.B.
A space for small group and "one on one" activities, which shall be readily accessible to the residents.

*8.4.B1. Space and equipment for carrying out each of the activities defined in the functional program.

8.4.B2. Resident toilet room(s) convenient to the area. Exception: Renovation projects need not comply with these requirements.

Nothing in these guidelines is intended to restrict a facility from providing additional square footage per resident beyond what is required herein for activities.

8.5 Rehabilitation Therapy

Each nursing facility which provides physical and/or occupational therapy services for rehabilitating long-term care residents shall have areas and equipment that conform to program intent. When the nursing facility is part of a general hospital or other facility, services may be shared as appropriate.

8.5.A. Physical and Occupational Therapy Provisions (Inpatient/Outpatient):

As a minimum, the following shall be located on-site, convenient for use:

8.5.A1. Space for files, records, and administrative activities.

8.5.A2. Provisions for wheelchair residents.

8.5.A3. Storage for supplies and equipment.

8.5.A4. Handwashing facilities within the therapy unit.

8.5.A5. Space and equipment for carrying out each of the types of therapy that may be prescribed.

8.5.A6. Provisions for resident privacy.

8.5.A7. Housekeeping rooms, in or near unit.

8.5.A8. Resident toilet room(s), usable by wheelchair residents.

8.5.B. Physical and Occupational Therapy for Outpatients
If the program includes outpatient treatment, additional provisions shall include:

8.5.B1. Convenient facility access usable by the disabled.

8.5.B2. Lockers for storing patients' clothing and personal effects.

8.5.B3. Outpatient facilities for dressing.

8.5.B4. Shower(s) for patients' use.

*8.6 Personal Services (Barber/Beauty) Areas

Facilities and equipment for resident hair care and grooming shall be provided separate from the resident rooms. These may be unisex and can be located adjacent to central resident activity areas, provided that location and scheduling preserve patient dignity.

*8.7 Subacute Care Facilities

8.8 Alzheimer's and Other Dementia Units

*8.8.A.
Safety: Safety concerns must be emphasized because of poor judgment inherent in those with dementia. Areas or pieces of furniture that could be hazardous to these residents should be eliminated or designed to minimize possible accidents.

8.8.A1.
Doors: The security of the resident shall be addressed through systems that secure the unit and comply with life safety codes.

8.8.A2.
Windows: May be operable, but must be secured, so residents cannot climb out.

*8.8.B.
Outdoor spaces: Outdoor gardens and lounge areas shall be available for residents of the Alzheimer's/Dementia resident unit.

*8.8.C.
Activities: Activity space for resident use in dementia programs shall be provided.

8.9 Dietary Facilities

The following services shall be provided:

8.9.A.
Food service facilities and equipment shall conform with these standards and other applicable food and sanitation codes and standards and shall provide food service for residents.

Food receiving, storage, and preparation areas shall facilitate quality control. Provision shall be made for transport of hot and cold foods, as required by the functional program. Separate dining areas shall be provided for staff and for residents. The design and location of dining facilities shall encourage resident use.

Facilities shall also be furnished to provide nourishments and snacks between scheduled meal service.

The dietary facility shall be easy to clean and to maintain in a sanitary condition.

8.9.B. Functional Elements

If the dietary department is on-site, the following facilities, in the size and number appropriate for the type of food service selected, shall be provided:

8.9.B1. A control station for receiving and controlling food supplies.

8.9.B2. Storage space, including cold storage, for at least a 4-day supply of food. (Facilities in remote areas may require proportionally more food storage facilities.)

8.9.B3. Food preparation facilities. Conventional food preparation systems require space and equipment for preparing, cooking, and baking. Convenience food service systems using frozen prepared meals, bulk packaged entrees, individual packaged portions, or those using contractual commissary services, require space and equipment for thawing, portioning, cooking, and/or baking.

8.9.B4. Handwashing facility(ies) located in the food preparation area.

8.9.B5. Facilities for assembly and distribution of patient meals.

8.9.B6. Separate dining spaces for residents and staff.

8.9.B7. Warewashing space located in a room or an alcove separate from the food preparation and serving area. Commercial-type warewashing equipment shall be provided. Space shall also be provided for receiving, scraping, sorting, and stacking soiled tableware and for transferring clean tableware to the using areas. Convenient handwashing facilities shall be available.

8.9.B8. Potwashing facilities.

8.9.B9. Storage areas and sanitizing facilities for cans, carts, and mobile-tray conveyors.

8.9.B10. Waste, storage, and recycling facilities (per local requirements) located in a separate room easily accessible to the outside for direct pickup or disposal.

8.9.B11. Office(s) or desk spaces for dietitian(s) and/or a dietary service manager.

8.9.B12. Toilet for dietary staff convenient to the kitchen area.

8.9.B13. A housekeeping room located within the dietary department. This shall include a floor receptor or service sink and storage space for housekeeping equipment and supplies.

8.9.B14. Ice-making facilities. These may be located in the food preparation area or in a separate room, shall be easily cleanable and convenient to the dietary function.

8.10. Administrative and Public Areas

The following shall be provided:

8.10.A. Vehicular Drop-Off and Pedestrian Entrance
This shall be at grade level, sheltered from inclement weather, and accessible to the disabled.

8.10.B. Administrative/Lobby Area

This shall include:

1. A counter or desk for reception and information.

2. Public waiting area(s).

3. Public toilet facilities.

4. Public telephone(s).

5. Drinking fountain(s).

8.10.C. General or Individual Office(s)
These shall be provided for business transactions, admissions, social services, medical and financial records, and administrative and professional staff. There shall be included provisions for private interviews.

8.10.D. Multipurpose Room(s)
There shall be a multipurpose room for conferences, meetings, and health education purposes as required by the functional program; it shall include provisions for the use of visual aids. One multipurpose room may be shared by several services.

8.10.E.
Clerical Files and Staff Office Space shall be provided as required by the functional program.

8.10.F. Supply room.
Space for storage of office equipment and supplies shall be provided as required by the functional program.

8.11 Linen Services

8.11.A. General
Each facility shall have provisions for storing and processing of clean and soiled/contaminated linen for appropriate resident care. Processing may be done within the facility, in a separate building on- or off-site, or in a commercial or shared laundry. At a minimum, the following elements shall be included:

1. Separate central or decentralized room(s) for receiving and holding soiled linen until ready for pickup or processing. Such room(s) shall have proper ventilation and exhaust.

2. A central, clean linen storage and issuing room(s), in addition to the linen storage required at individual resident units.

3. Provisions shall be made for parking of clean and soiled linen carts separately and out of traffic and for cleaning of linen carts on premises (or exchange carts off premises).

4. Handwashing facilities in each area where unbagged, soiled linen is handled.

8.11.B. Off-Site Processing
If linen is processed off-site or in a separate building on-site, provisions shall also be made for:

1. A service entrance, protected from inclement weather, for loading and unloading of linen. This can be shared with other services and serve as the loading dock for the facility.

2. Control station for pickup and receiving. This can be shared with other services and serve as the receiving and pickup point for the facility.

8.11.C. On-Site Processing

If linen is processed in a laundry facility within the facility, the following shall be provided in addition to the elements required by Section 8.12.B:

1. A receiving, holding, and sorting room for control and distribution of soiled linen. Discharge from soiled linen chutes may be received within this room or in a separate room adjacent to it.

2. Washers/extractors located between the soiled linen receiving and clean processing areas. Personal laundry, if decentralized, may be handled within one room or rooms, so long as there are separate, defined areas for handling clean and soiled laundry.

3. Storage for laundry supplies.

5. Linen inspection and mending area.

6. Arrangement of equipment that will permit an orderly work flow and minimize cross-traffic that might mix clean and soiled operations.

8.12 Housekeeping Rooms

Housekeeping rooms shall be provided throughout the facility as required to maintain a clean and sanitary environment. Each shall contain a floor receptor or service sink and storage space for housekeeping equipment and supplies. There shall be at least one housekeeping room for each floor.

8.13 Engineering Service and Equipment Areas

The following shall be provided as necessary for effective service and maintenance functions:

8.13.A. Room(s) or separate building(s) for boilers, mechanical, and electrical equipment.

8.13.B. Provisions for protected storage of facility drawings, records, manuals, etc.

8.13.C. General maintenance area for repair and maintenance.

8.13.D. Storage room for building maintenance supplies. Storage for solvents and flammable liquids shall comply with applicable NFPA codes.

8.13.E.
Yard equipment and supply storage areas shall be located so that equipment may be moved directly to the exterior.

8.13.F.
Loading dock, receiving and breakout area(s), if required by the functional program. These may be shared with other services.

8.13.G.
General storage space(s) shall be provided for furniture and equipment such as intravenous stands, inhalators, air mattresses, walkers, etc., medical supplies, housekeeping supplies and equipment.

*8.14 General Standards for Details and Finishes

Resident facilities require features that encourage ambulation of long-term residents. Signage and wayfinding features shall be provided to aid self-ambulating residents and avoid confusing or disorienting them. Potential hazards to residents, such as sharp corners, slippery floors, loose carpets, and hot surfaces should be avoided.

Renovations shall not diminish the level of compliance with these standards below that which existed prior to the renovation. However, features in excess of those for new constructions are not required to be maintained in the completed renovation.

8.14.A. Details

8.14.A1. The placement of drinking fountains, public telephones, and vending machines shall not restrict corridor traffic or reduce the corridor width below the minimum stipulated in NFPA 101.

8.14.A2. Doors to all rooms containing bathtubs, sitz baths, showers, and toilets for resident use shall be hinged, sliding, or folding.

8.14.A3. Windows and outer doors that may be left open shall have insect screens.

8.14.A4. Resident rooms or suites in new construction shall have window(s). Operable windows or vents that open from the inside shall be restricted to inhibit possible resident escape or suicide. Windows shall have sills located above grade, but no higher than 36 inches (91 centimeters) above the finished floor.

*8.14.A5. Glazing in doors, sidelights, borrowed lights, and windows where glazing is less than 18 inches (46 centimeters) from the floor shall be constructed of safety glass, wire glass, or plastic glazing material that resists breaking and creates no dangerous cutting edges when broken. Similar materials shall be used in wall openings in activity areas (such as recreation rooms and exercise rooms) if permitted by local requirements. If doors are provided for shower and tub enclosures glazing shall be safety glass or plastic.

8.14.A6. Thresholds and expansion joint covers shall be designed to facilitate use of wheelchairs and carts and to prevent tripping.

*8.14.A7. Grab bars shall be installed in all resident toilets, showers, tubs, and sitz baths. For wall-mounted grab bars, a minimum 1½ inch (3.81 centimeters) clearance from walls is required. Bars, including those which are part of fixtures such as soap dishes, shall have the strength to sustain a concentrated load of 250 pounds (113.4 kilograms).

*8.14.A8. Handrails shall be provided on both sides of all corridors normally used by residents. A minimum clearance of 1½ inches (3.81 centimeters) shall be provided between the handrail and the wall. Rail ends shall be finished to minimize potential for personal injury.

8.14.A9. Handwashing facilities shall be constructed with sufficient clearance for blade-type operating handles.

8.14.A10. Lavatories, and handwashing facilities and handrails which a resident could use for support shall be securely anchored.

8.14.A11. Each resident handwashing facility shall have a mirror. Mirror placement shall allow for convenient use by both wheelchair occupants and/or ambulatory persons. Tops and bottoms may be at levels usable by individuals either sitting or standing, or additional mirrors may be provided for wheelchair occupants. One separate full-length mirror may serve for wheelchair occupants.

8.14.A12. Provisions for hand drying shall be included at all handwashing facilities. These shall be paper or cloth towels enclosed to protect against dust or soil and to ensure single-unit dispensing.

8.14.A13. The minimum ceiling height shall be 7 feet 10 inches (2.39 meters) with the following exceptions:

a. Boiler rooms shall have ceiling clearances of at least 2 feet 6 inches (76.20 centimeters) above the main boiler header and connecting pipe.

b. Rooms containing ceiling-mounted equipment shall have the required ceiling height to ensure proper functioning of that equipment.

c. Ceilings in corridors, storage rooms, and toilet rooms shall be at least 7 feet 8 inches (2.34 meters). Ceilings in normally unoccupied spaces may be reduced to 7 feet (2.13 meters).

d. Building components and suspended tracks, rails, and pipes located along the path of normal traffic shall be not less than 7 feet (2.13 meters) above the floor.

e. In buildings being renovated, it is desirable to maintain minimum ceiling heights per subparagraphs a through d above. However, in no case shall ceiling heights be reduced more than 4 inches (10.16 centimeters) below the minimum requirement for new construction.

f. Architecturally framed and trimmed openings in corridors and rooms shall be permitted, provided a minimum clear opening height of 7 feet (2.13 meters) is maintained.

8.14.A14. Rooms containing heat-producing equipment (such as boiler rooms, heater rooms, and laundries) shall be insulated and ventilated to prevent the floors of occupied areas overhead and the adjacent walls from exceeding a temperature of 10oFahrenheit (6oC) above the ambient room temperature of such occupied areas.

8.15 Finishes

8.15.A.
Cubicle curtains and draperies shall be noncombustible or flame-retardant as prescribed in both the large- and small-scale tests in NFPA 701.

8.15.B.
Materials provided by the facility for finishes and furnishings, including mattresses and upholstery, shall comply with NFPA 101.

8.15.C.
Floor materials shall be readily cleanable and appropriate for the location. Floors in areas used for food preparation and assembly shall be water-resistant. Floor surfaces, including tile joints, shall be resistant to food acids. In all areas subject to frequent wet-cleaning methods, floor

materials shall not be physically affected by germicidal cleaning solutions. Floors subject to traffic while wet (such as shower and bath areas, kitchens, and similar work areas) shall have a slip-resistant surface. Carpet and padding in resident areas shall be glued down or stretched taut and free of loose edges or wrinkles that might create hazards or interfere with the operation of wheelchairs, walkers, wheeled carts, etc.

8.15.D.
Wall bases in areas subject to routine wet cleaning shall be coved and tightly sealed.

8.15.E.
Wall finishes shall be washable and, if near plumbing fixtures, shall be smooth and moisture-resistant. Finish, trim, walls, and floor constructions in dietary and food storage areas shall be free from rodent- and insect-harboring spaces.

8.15.F.
Floor and wall openings for pipes, ducts, and conduits shall be tightly sealed to resist fire and smoke and to minimize entry of pests. Joints of structural elements shall be similarly sealed.

8.15.G.
The finishes of all exposed ceilings and ceiling structures in resident rooms and staff work areas shall be readily cleanable with routine housekeeping equipment. Finished ceilings shall be provided in dietary and other areas where dust fallout might create a problem.

8.15.H.
Directional and identification signage shall comply with ADA guidelines.

8.16 Construction Features

All parts of the nursing facility shall be designed and constructed to sustain dead and live loads in accordance with local and national building codes and accepted engineering practices and standards, including requirements for seismic forces and applicable sections of NFPA 101.

8.17 Reserved

8.18 Reserved

8.19 Reserved

8.20 Reserved

8.21 Reserved

8.22 Reserved

8.23 Reserved

8.24 Reserved

8.25 Reserved

8.26 Reserved

8.27 Reserved

8.28 Reserved

8.29 Reserved

8.30 Special Systems

8.30.A General

8.30.A1. Prior to acceptance of the facility, all special systems shall be tested and operated to demonstrate to the owner or designated representative that the installation and performance of these systems conform to design intent. Test results shall be documented for maintenance files.

8.30.A2. Upon completion of the special systems equipment installation contract, the owner shall be furnished with a complete set of manufacturers' operating, maintenance, and preventive maintenance instructions, a parts list, and complete procurement information including equipment numbers and descriptions. Operating staff persons shall also be provided with instructions for proper operation of systems and equipment. Required information shall include all safety or code ratings as needed.

8.30.A3. Insulation shall be provided surrounding special system equipment to conserve energy, protect personnel, and reduce noise.

8.30.B Elevators

8.30.B1. All buildings having resident use areas on more than one floor shall have electric or hydraulic elevator(s). Installation and testing of elevators shall comply with ANSI/ASME A17.1 (for new construction) or ANSI/ASME 17.3 (for existing buildings). (See ASCE 7-93 for seismic design and control systems requirements for elevators.)

a. Engineered traffic studies are recommended, but in their absence the following guidelines for minimum number of elevators shall apply (**Note:** these standards may be inadequate for moving large numbers of people in a short time; adjustments should be made as appropriate):

i. At least one hospital-type elevator shall be installed where residents are housed on any floor other than the main entrance floor.

ii. When 60 to 200 residents are housed on floors other than the main entrance floor, at least two elevators, one of which shall be of the hospital-type, shall be installed.

iii. When 201 to 350 residents are housed on floors other than main entrance floor, at least three elevators, one of which shall be of the hospital-type, shall be installed.

iv. For facilities with more than 350 residents housed above the main entrance floor, the number of elevators shall be determined from a facility plan study and from the estimated vertical transportation requirements.

v. When the nursing facility is part of a general hospital, elevators may be shared and the standards of Section 7.30 shall apply.

*8.30.B2. Cars of hospital-type elevators shall have inside dimensions that accommodate a resident bed with attendants. The clear inside dimension of such cars shall be at least 5 feet (1.52 meters) wide by 7 feet 6 inches (2.29 meters) deep. Car doors shall have a clear opening of not less than 3 feet 8 inches (1.12 meters). Other elevators required for passenger service shall be constructed to accommodate wheelchairs.

8.30.B3. Elevators shall be equipped with an automatic two-way leveling device with an accuracy of $\pm \frac{1}{4}$ inch (.64 centimeter).

8.30.C. Waste Processing Service

Facilities shall be provided for sanitary storage and treatment or disposal of waste and recyclables using techniques and capacities acceptable to the appropriate health and environmental authorities.

8.31 Mechanical Standards

8.31.A. General

8.31.A1. The mechanical system shall be subject to general review for operational efficiency and appropriate life-cycle cost. Details for cost-effective implementation of design features are interrelated and too numerous (as well as too basic) to list individually. Recognized engineering procedures shall be followed for the most economical and effective results. A well-designed system can generally achieve energy efficiency with minimal additional cost and simultaneously provide improved resident comfort. In no case shall resident care or safety be sacrificed for conservation.

8.31.A2. Facility design considerations shall include site, building, location, climate, orientation, configuration, and thermal requirements.

8.31.A3. As appropriate, controls for air-handling systems shall be designed with an economizer cycle to use outside air for cooling and/or heating.

8.31.A4. To maintain asepsis control, airflow supply and exhaust should generally be controlled to ensure movement of air from "clean" to "less clean" areas.

8.31.A5. Supply and return mains and risers for cooling, heating, and steam systems shall be equipped with valves to isolate the various sections of each system. Each piece of equipment shall have valves at the supply and return ends.

8.31.B. Thermal and Acoustical Insulation

8.31.B1. Insulation within the building shall be provided to conserve energy, protect personnel, prevent vapor condensation, and reduce noise.

8.31.B2. Insulation on cold surfaces shall include an exterior vapor barrier. (Insulating material that will not absorb or transmit moisture will not require a separate vapor barrier.)

8.31.B3. Insulation, including finishes and adhesives on the exterior surfaces of ducts, piping, and equipment, shall have a flame-spread rating of 25 or less and a smoke-developed rating of 50 or less as determined by an independent testing laboratory in accordance with NFPA 255.

8.31.B4. If duct lining is used, it shall be coated and sealed and shall meet ASTM C1071. These linings (including coatings, adhesives, and exterior surface insulation of pipes and ducts in spaces used as air supply plenums) shall have a flame-spread rating of 25 or less and a smoke-developed rating of 50 or less, as determined by an independent testing laboratory in accordance with NFPA 255. Duct lining may not be installed within 15 feet (4.57 meters) downstream of humidifiers.

8.31.B5. In facilities undergoing major renovations, existing accessible insulation shall be inspected, repaired, and/or replaced as appropriate.

8.31.C. Steam and Hot Water Systems

8.31.C1. Boilers shall have the capacity, based on the net ratings published by the Hydronics Institute or another acceptable national standard, to supply not less than 70 percent of the normal requirements of all systems and equipment. Their number and arrangement shall accommodate facility needs despite the breakdown or routine maintenance of any one boiler. The capacity of the remaining boiler(s) shall be sufficient to provide hot water service for clinical, dietary, and resident use; steam for dietary purposes; and heating for general resident rooms. However, reserve capacity for facility space heating is not required in geographic areas where a design dry-bulb temperature of 25° Fahrenheit (-4°C) or more represents not less than 99 percent of the total hours in any one heating month as noted in ASHRAE's Handbook of Fundamentals, under the "Table for Climatic Conditions for the United States."

8.31.C2. Boiler accessories, including feed pumps, heat-circulating pumps, condensate return pumps, fuel oil pumps, and waste heat boilers, shall be connected and installed to provide both normal and standby service.

8.31.D. Air Conditioning, Heating, and Ventilation Systems

***8.31.D1.** The ventilation rates shown in Table 6, as applicable, shall be used only as minimum standards; they do not preclude the use of higher rates as appropriate. All rooms and areas in the facility shall have provision for positive ventilation. Though natural window ventilation may be utilized where weather and outside air quality permit, use of mechanical ventilation should be considered for interior areas and during periods of temperature extremes. Non-central air-handling systems, e.g., through-the-wall fan coil units, may be utilized. Fans serving exhaust systems shall be located at the discharge end and shall be readily serviceable. Exhaust systems may be combined to enhance the efficiency of recovery devices required for energy conservation.

8.31.D2. When appropriate, mechanical ventilation should employ an economizer cycle that uses outside air to reduce heating-and-cooling-system loads. Filtering will be necessary when outside air is used as part of the mechanical ventilation system. Innovative design that provides for additional energy conservation while meeting the intent of these standards for acceptable resident care should be considered.

8.31.D3. Fresh air intakes shall be located at least 25 feet (7.62 meters) from exhaust outlets of ventilating systems, combustion equipment stacks, medical-surgical vacuum systems, plumbing vents, or areas that may collect vehicular exhaust or other noxious fumes. (Prevailing winds and/or proximity to other structures may require greater clearances.) The bottom of outdoor air intakes serving central ventilating systems shall be as high as practical, but at least 6 feet (1.83 meters) above ground level, or, if installed above roof, 3 feet (0.91 meter) above roof level. Exhaust outlets from areas that may be contaminated shall be above roof level, arranged to minimize recirculation of exhaust air into the building.

8.31.D4. The ventilation systems shall be designed and balanced to provide directional flow as shown in Table 6.

8.31.D5. All central ventilation or air conditioning systems shall be equipped with filters with efficiencies equal to, or greater than, those specified in Table 7. Filter efficiencies, tested in accordance with ASHRAE Standard 52-92, shall be average. Filter frames shall be durable and proportioned to provide an airtight fit with the enclosing ductwork. All joints between filter segments and the enclosing ductwork shall have gaskets or seals to provide a positive seal against air leakage.

8.31.D6. Air-handling duct systems shall meet the requirements of NFPA 90A and those contained herein.

8.31.D7. Fire and smoke dampers shall be constructed, located, and installed in accordance with the requirements of NFPA 101, 90A, and the specific damper's listing requirements. Fans, dampers, and detectors shall be interconnected so that damper activation will not damage ducts. Maintenance access shall be provided at all dampers. All damper locations should be shown on drawings. Dampers should be activated by fire or smoke sensor, not by fan cutoff alone.

Switching systems for restarting fans may be installed for fire department use in evacuating smoke after a fire has been controlled. However, provisions should be made to avoid possible damage to the system because of closed dampers.

When smoke partitions are required, heating, ventilating, and air conditioning zones shall be coordinated with compartmentation insofar as practical to minimize the need to penetrate fire and smoke partitions.

***8.31.D8.** Non-central air-handling systems, e.g., through-the-wall fan coil units, shall be equipped with permanent (cleanable) or replaceable filters rated at a minimum efficiency of 68 percent arrestance per ASHRAE Test Methods Standard 52.1-92.

8.31.D9. Rooms with fuel-fired equipment shall be provided with sufficient outdoor air to maintain equipment combustion rates and to limit workstation temperatures.

8.31.E. Plumbing and Other Piping Systems
Unless otherwise specified herein, all plumbing systems shall be designed and installed in accordance with the *National Standard Plumbing Code,* chapter 14, Medical Care Facility Plumbing Equipment.

8.31.E1. The following standards shall apply to plumbing fixtures:

a. The material used for plumbing fixtures shall be non-absorptive.

b. Water spouts used in lavatories and sinks shall have clearances adequate to avoid contaminating utensils and the contents of carafes, etc.

c. All fixtures used by staff and all lavatories used by food handlers shall be trimmed with valves that can be operated without hands (single-lever devices may be used). Blade handles used for this purpose shall not exceed 4½ inches (11.43 centimeters) in length. Handles on scrub sinks and clinical sinks shall be at least 6 inches (15.24 centimeters) long.

d. Clinical sinks shall have an integral trap wherein the upper portion of the water trap provides a visible seal.

e. Showers and tubs shall have a slip-resistant surface.

8.31.E2. The following standards shall apply to potable water supply systems:

a. Systems shall be designed to supply water at sufficient pressure to operate all fixtures and equipment during maximum demand. Supply capacity for hot- and cold-water piping shall be determined on the basis of fixture units, using recognized engineering standards. When the ratio of plumbing fixtures to occupants is proportionally more than required by the building occupancy and is in excess of 1,000 plumbing fixture units, a diversity factor is permitted.

b. Each water service main, branch main, riser, and branch to a group of fixtures shall have valves. Stop valves shall be provided for each fixture. Appropriate panels for access shall be provided at all valves where required.

c. Backflow preventers (vacuum breakers) shall be installed on hose bibbs and supply nozzles used for connection of hoses or tubing in housekeeping sinks, bed-pan-flushing attachments, etc.

d. Potable water storage vessels (hot and cold) not intended for constant use shall not be installed.

8.31.E3. The following standards shall apply to hot water systems:

a. The water-heating system shall have sufficient supply capacity at the temperatures and amounts indicated in Table 8. Water temperature is measured at the point of use or inlet to the equipment.

b. Hot-water distribution systems serving resident care areas shall be under constant recirculation to provide continuous hot water at each hot water outlet. The temperature of hot water for showers and bathing shall be appropriate for comfortable use but shall not exceed 110° Fahrenheit (43°C).

8.31.E4. The following standards shall apply to drainage systems:

a. Insofar as possible, drainage piping shall not be installed within the ceiling or exposed in food preparation centers, food serving facilities, food storage areas, central services, electronic data processing areas, electric closets, and other sensitive areas. Where exposed, overhead drain piping in these areas is unavoidable, special provisions shall be made to protect the space below from leakage, condensation, or dust particles.

b. Building sewers shall discharge into community sewerage. Where such a system is not available, the facility shall treat its sewage in accordance with local and state regulations.

c. Kitchen grease traps shall be located and arranged to permit easy access.

8.31.E5. Any installation of nonflammable medical gas, air, or clinical vacuum systems shall comply with the requirements of NFPA 99. When any piping or supply of medical gases is installed, altered, or augmented, the altered zone shall be tested and certified as required by NFPA 99.

8.31.E6. All piping, except control-line tubing, shall be identified. All valves shall be tagged, and a valve schedule shall be provided to the facility owner for permanent record and reference.

8.32 Electrical Standards

8.32.A. General

8.32.A1. All material and equipment, including conductors, controls, and signaling devices, shall be installed to provide a complete electrical system in accordance with NFPA 70 and NFPA 99.

A.32.A2. All electrical installations and systems shall be tested to verify that the equipment has been installed and that it operates as designed.

8.32.A3. Electrical systems for nursing facilities shall comply with applicable sections of NFPA 70.

8.32.A4. Lighting shall be engineered to the specific application.

*a. The Illuminating Engineering Society of North America (IES) has developed recommended minimum lighting levels for nursing facilities.

*b. Approaches to buildings and parking lots, and all occupied spaces within buildings shall have fixtures for lighting. Consideration shall be given to contrast in lighting levels.

*c. Resident rooms shall have general lighting and night lighting. A reading light shall be provided for each resident. Reading light controls shall be readily accessible to residents. At least one night light fixture in each resident room shall be controlled at the room entrance. All light controls in resident areas shall be quiet-operating.

d. Resident unit corridors shall have general illumination with provisions for reducing light levels at night.

8.32.A5. Receptacles (Convenience Outlets)

a. Each resident room shall have duplex-grounded receptacles. There shall be one at each side of the head of each bed and one on every other wall. Receptacles may be omitted from exterior walls where construction makes installation impractical.

b. Duplex-grounded receptacles for general use shall be installed approximately 50 feet (15.24 meters) apart in all corridors and within 25 feet (7.62 meters) of corridor ends.

c. Electrical receptacle coverplates or electrical receptacles supplied from the emergency system shall be distinctively colored or marked for identification. If color is used for identification purposes, the same color should be used throughout the facility.

d. Ground-fault-interrupters shall comply with NFPA 70.

8.32.B. Reserved

8.32.C. Reserved

8.32.D. Reserved

8.32.E. Reserved

8.32.F. Reserved

8.32.G. Nurse/Staff Call System

A nurses/staff call system shall be provided. Each bed location and/or resident shall be provided with a call device. Two call devices serving adjacent beds or residents may be served by one calling station. Calls shall be initiated by a resident activating either a call device attached to a resident's calling station, or a portable device which sends a call signal to the calling station and shall either:

(a) Activate a visual signal in the corridor at the resident's door or other appropriate location. In multi-corridor or cluster resident units, additional visual signals shall be installed at corridor intersections; or

(b) Activate a pager worn by a staff member, identifying the specific resident and/or room from which the call has been placed.

An emergency call system shall be provided at each resident toilet, bath, sitz bath, and shower room. This system shall be accessible to a resident lying on the floor. Inclusion of a pull cord or portable radio frequency pushbutton will satisfy this standard.

The emergency call system shall be designed so that a call activated by a resident will initiate a signal distinct from the regular staff call system and that can be turned off only at the resident's location. The signal shall activate an annunciator panel or screen at the staff work area or other appropriate location, and either a visual signal in the corridor at the resident's door or other appropriate location, or a staff pager indicating the calling resident's name and/or room location, and at other areas defined by the functional program.

Alternate technologies can be considered for emergency or nurse call systems. If radio frequency systems are used, consideration should be given to electromagnetic compatibility between internal and external sources.

8.32.H. Emergency Electrical Service

8.32.H1 As a minimum, nursing facilities or sections thereof shall have emergency electrical systems as required in NFPA 101 and Chapter 16 of NFPA 99.

8.32.H2 When the nursing facility is a distinct part of an acute-care hospital, it may use the emergency generator system for required emergency lighting and power, if such sharing does not reduce hospital services. Life support systems and their respective areas shall be subject to applicable standards of Section 7.32.

8.32.H3 An emergency electrical source shall provide lighting and/or power during an interruption of the normal electric supply. Where stored fuel is required, storage capacity shall permit continuous operation for at least 24 hours. Fuel storage for electricity generation shall be separate from heating fuels. If the use of heating fuel for diesel engines is considered after the required 24-hour supply has been exhausted, positive valving and filtration shall be provided to avoid entry of water and/or contaminants.

8.32.H4. Local codes and regulations may have additional requirements.

8.32.H5. Exhaust systems (including locations, mufflers, and vibration isolators) for internal combustion engines shall be designed and installed to minimize objectionable noise. Where a generator is routinely used to reduce peak loads, protection of patient areas from excessive noise may become a critical issue.

8.32.I Fire Alarm System
Fire alarm and detection systems shall be provided in compliance with NFPA 101 and NFPA 72.

8.32.J Telecommunication and Information Systems

Table 6

Pressure Relationships and Ventilation of Certain Areas of Nursing Facilities[1]

Area designation	Air movement relationship to adjacent area[2]	Minimum air changes of outdoor air per hour[3]	Minimum total air changes per hour[4]	All air exhausted directly to outdoors[5]	Recirculated by means of room units[6]	Relative humidity[7] (%)	Design temperature[8] (degrees F/C)
Resident room	—	2	2	—	—	[9]	70-75 (21–24)
Resident unit corridor	—	—	2	—	—	[9]	—
Toilet Room	In	—	10	Yes	—	—	—
Protective environment rooms, if provided[10]	Out	2	12	—	No	—	75 (24)
Airborne infectious isolation rooms, if provided	In	2	12	Yes	No	—	70-75 (21–24)
Isolation alcoves or anterooms, if provided[11]	In/Out	—	10	Yes	No	—	—
Dining rooms	—	2	2	—	75		
Activity rooms, if provided	—	2	2	—	—	—	—
Physical therapy	In	2	6	—	—	—	75 (24)
Occupational therapy	In	2	6	—	—	—	75 (24)
Soiled workroom or soiled holding	In	2	10	Yes	No	—	—
Clean workroom or clean holding	Out	2	4	—	—	(Max) 70	75 (24)
Sterilizer exhaust room	In	—	10	Yes	No	—	—
Linen and trash chute room, if provided	In	—	10	Yes	No	—	—
Laundry, general, if provided	—	2	10	Yes	No	—	—
Soiled linen sorting and storage	In	—	10	Yes	No	—	—
Clean linen storage	Out	—	2	Yes	No	—	—
Food preparation facilities[12]	—	2	10	Yes	Yes	—	—
Dietary warewashing	In	—	10	Yes	Yes	—	—
Dietary storage areas	—	—	2	Yes	No	—	—
Housekeeping rooms	In	—	10	Yes	No	—	—
Bathing rooms	In	—	10	Yes	No	—	75 (24)

(continued on next page)

Notes

1 The ventilation rates in this table cover ventilation for comfort, as well as for asepsis and odor control in areas of nursing facilities that directly affect resident care and are determined based on nursing facilities being predominantly "No Smoking" facilities. Where smoking may be allowed, ventilation rates will need adjustments. Areas where specific ventilation rates are not given in the table shall be ventilated in accordance with ASHRAE Standard 62, *Ventilation for Acceptable Indoor Air Quality,* and ASHRAE *Handbook of Applications.* OSHA standards and/or NIOSH criteria require special ventilation requirements for employee health and safety within nursing facilities.

2 Design of the ventilation system shall, insofar as possible, provide that air movement is from "clean to less clean" areas. However, continuous compliance may be impractical with full utilization of some forms of variable air volume and load shedding systems that may be used for energy conservation. Areas that do require positive and continuous control are noted with "Out" or "In" to indicate the required direction of air movement in relation to the space named. Rate of air movement may, of course, be varied as needed within the limits required for positive control. Where indication of air movement direction is enclosed in parentheses, continuous directional control is required only when the specialized equipment or device is in use or where room use may otherwise compromise the intent of movement from clean to less clean. Air movement for rooms with dashes and nonpatient areas may vary as necessary to satisfy the requirements of those spaces. Additional adjustments may be needed when space is unused or unoccupied and air systems are deenergized or reduced.

3 To satisfy exhaust needs, replacement air from outside is necessary. Table 6 does not attempt to describe specific amounts of outside air to be supplied to individual spaces except for certain areas such as those listed. Distribution of the outside air, added to the system to balance required exhaust, shall be as required by good engineering practice.

4 Number of air changes may be reduced when the room is unoccupied if provisions are made to ensure that the number of air changes indicated is reestablished any time the space is being utilized. Adjustments shall include provisions so that the direction of air movement shall remain the same when the number of air changes is reduced. Areas not indicated as having continuous directional control may have ventilation systems shut down when space is unoccupied and ventilation is not otherwise needed.

5 Air from areas with contamination and/or odor problems shall be exhausted to the outside and not recirculated to other areas. Note that individual circumstances may require special consideration for air exhaust to outside.

6 Because of cleaning difficulty and potential for buildup of contamination, recirculating room units shall not be used in areas marked "No." Isolation rooms may be ventilated by reheat induction units in which only the primary air supplied from a central system passes through the reheat unit. Gravity-type heating or cooling units such as radiators or convectors shall not be used in special care areas.

*7 The ranges listed are the minimum and maximum limits where control is specifically needed. See A8.31.D for additional information.

8 When temperature ranges are indicated, the systems shall be capable of maintaining the rooms at any point within the range. A single figure indicates a heating or cooling capacity of at least the indicated temperature. This is usually applicable where residents may be undressed and require a warmer environment. Nothing in these guidelines shall be construed as precluding the use of temperatures lower than those noted when the residents' comfort and medical conditions make lower temperatures desirable. Unoccupied areas such as storage rooms shall have temperatures appropriate for the function intended.

*9 See A8.31.D1.

*10 The protective environment airflow design specifications protect the patient from common environmental airborne infectious microbes (i.e., Aspergillus spores). These special ventilation areas shall be designed to provide directed airflow from the cleanest patient care area to less clean areas. These rooms shall be protected with HEPA filters at 99.97 percent efficiency for a 0.3 µm sized particle in the supply airstream. These interrupting filters protect patient rooms from maintenance-derived release of environmental microbes from the ventilation system components. Recirculation HEPA filters can be used to increase the equivalent room air exchanges. Constant volume airflow is required for consistent ventilation for the protected environment. If the facility determines that airborne infection isolation is necessary for protective environment patients, an anteroom shall be provided. Rooms with reversible airflow provisions for the purpose of switching between protective isolation and airborne infection isolation functions are not acceptable.

11 The infectious disease isolation room described in these guidelines is to be used for isolating the airborne spread of infectious diseases, such as measles, varicella, or tuberculosis. The design of airborne infection isolation (AII) rooms should include the provision for normal patient care during periods not requiring isolation precautions. Supplemental recirculating devices may be used in the patient room, to increase the equivalent room air exchanges; however, such recirculating devices do not provide the outside air requirements. Air may be recirculated within individual isolation rooms if HEPA filters are used. Rooms with reversible airflow provisions for the purpose of switching between protective isolation and airborne infection isolation functions are not acceptable.

12 Food preparation facilities shall have ventilation systems whose air supply mechanisms are interfaced appropriately with exhaust hood controls or relief vents so that exfiltration or infiltration to or from exit corridors does not compromise the exit corridor restrictions of NFPA 90A, the pressure requirements of NFPA 96, or the maximum defined in the table. The number of air changes may be reduced or varied to any extent required for odor control when the space is not in use.

Table 7

Filter Efficiencies for Central Ventilation and Air Conditioning Systems in Nursing Facilities

Area Designation	Minimum number of filter beds	Filter efficiencies (%)	
		Filter bed no. 1	Filter bed no. 2
All areas for inpatient care, treatment, and/or diagnosis, and those areas providing direct service or clean supplies	2	30	80
Administrative, bulk storage, soiled holding, laundries, food preparation areas	1	30	

Note: The filtration efficiency ratings are based on dust spot efficiency per ASHRAE 52–92.

Table 8

Hot Water Use—Nursing Facilities

	Resident Care Areas	Dietary[†]	Laundry
Liters per second per bed*	0.0033	0.0020	0.0021
Gallons per hour per bed*	3	2	2
Temperature (Centigrade)**	35–43	60	60**
Temperature (Fahrenheit)**	95–110 (max.)	140 (min.)	140 (min.)**

[†] Provisions may be made to provide 180° Fahrenheit (82°C) rinse water at warewasher (may be by separate booster).

*Quantities indicated for design demand of hot water are for general reference minimums and shall not substitute for accepted engineering design procedures using actual number and types of fixtures to be installed. Design will also be affected by temperatures of cold water used for mixing, length of run, and insulation relative to heat loss, etc. As an example, total quantity of hot water needed will be less when temperature available at the outlet is very nearly that of the source tank and the cold water used for tempering is relatively warm.

**However, it is emphasized that this does not imply that all water used would be at this temperature. Water temperatures required for acceptable laundry results will vary according to type of cycle, time of operation, and formula of soap and bleach as well as type and degree of soil. Lower temperatures may be adequate for most procedures in many facilities but higher temperatures should be available when needed for special conditions. Minimum laundry temperatures are for central laundries only.

9. OUTPATIENT FACILITIES

9.1 General

9.1.A. Section Applicability

This section applies to the outpatient unit in a hospital or freestanding facility within a nonmedical facility or part of a health maintenance organization (HMO) or other health service. This section does not apply to the offices of private-practice physicians in commercial office space and should not be applied to such offices in ancillary outpatient facilities.

The general standards set forth in Sections 9.1 and 9.2 apply to each of the items below. Additions and/or modifications shall be made as described for the specific facility type.

Specialty facilities such as those for renal dialysis, cancer treatment, mental health, rehabilitation, etc., have needs that are not addressed here. They must satisfy additional conditions to meet respective programs' standards.

Specifically described are:

9.1.A1. Primary Care Outpatient Center (Section 9.3).

9.1.A2. The Small Primary (Neighborhood) Outpatient Facility (Section 9.4).

9.1.A3. The Outpatient Surgical Facility (Section 9.5).

9.1.A4. The Freestanding Emergency Facility (Section 9.6).

9.1.A5. Freestanding Birthing Center (Section 9.7).

9.1.B. Outpatient Facility Classification

Except for the emergency unit, the outpatient facilities described herein are used primarily by patients capable of traveling into, around, and out of the facility unassisted. This includes the disabled confined to wheelchairs. Occasional facility use by stretcher patients should not be used as a basis for more restrictive institutional occupancy classifications.

Facilities shall comply with the "Ambulatory Health Care Centers" section of NFPA 101, in addition to details herein, where patients incapable of self-preservation or those receiving inhalation anesthesia are treated. The "Business Occupancy" section of NFPA 101 applies to other types of outpatient facilities. Outpatient units that are part of another facility may be subject to the additional requirements of the other occupancy.

References are made to Section 7, General Hospital, for certain service spaces such as the operating rooms of the outpatient surgical unit. Those references are intended only for the specific areas indicated.

9.1.C. Facility Access

Where the outpatient unit is part of another facility, separation and access shall be maintained as described in NFPA 101. Building entrances used to reach the outpatient services shall be at grade level, clearly marked, and located so that patients need not go through other activity areas. (Lobbies of multi-occupancy buildings may be shared.) Design shall preclude unrelated traffic within the unit.

9.1.D. Functional Program Provision

Each project sponsor shall provide a functional program for the facility. (See Section 1.1.F.)

9.1.E. Shared/Purchased Services

When services are shared or purchased, space and equipment should be modified or eliminated to avoid unnecessary duplication.

9.1.F. Location

Community outpatient units shall be conveniently accessible to patients and staff via available public transportation.

9.1.G. Parking

In the absence of a formal parking study, parking for outpatient facilities shall be provided at the rate noted for each type of unit. On-street parking, if available, may satisfy part of this requirement unless described otherwise. If the facility is located in a densely populated area where a large percentage of patients arrive as pedestrians; or if adequate public parking is available nearby; or if the facility is conveniently accessible via public transportation, adjustments to this standard may be made with approval of the appropriate authorities.

9.1.H. Privacy for Patients

Each facility design shall ensure patient audible and visual privacy and dignity during interviews, examinations, treatment, and recovery.

9.2 Common Elements for Outpatient Facilities

The following shall apply to each outpatient facility described herein with additions and/or modifications as noted for each specific type. Special consideration shall be given to needs of children for pediatric services.

9.2.A. Administration and Public Areas

9.2.A1. Entrance. Located at grade level and able to accommodate wheelchairs.

9.2.A2. Public services shall include:

a. Conveniently accessible wheelchair storage.

b. A reception and information counter or desk.

c. Waiting space(s). Where an organized pediatric service is part of the outpatient facility, provisions shall be made for separating pediatric and adult patients.

d. Conveniently accessible public toilets.

e. Conveniently accessible public telephone(s).

f. Conveniently accessible drinking fountain(s).

9.2.A3. Interview space(s) for private interviews related to social service, credit, etc., shall be provided.

9.2.A4. General or individual office(s) for business transactions, records, administrative, and professional staffs shall be provided.

9.2.A5. Clerical space or rooms for typing, clerical work, and filing, separated from public areas for confidentiality, shall be provided.

9.2.A6. Multipurpose room(s) equipped for visual aids shall be provided for conferences, meetings, and health education purposes.

9.2.A7. Special storage for staff personal effects with locking drawers or cabinets (may be individual desks or cabinets) shall be provided. Such storage shall be near individual workstations and staff controlled.

9.2.A8. General storage facilities for supplies and equipment shall be provided as needed for continuing operation.

9.2.B. Clinical Facilities

As needed, the following elements shall be provided for clinical services to satisfy the functional program:

9.2.B1. General-purpose examination room(s). For medical, obstetrical, and similar examinations, rooms shall have a minimum floor area of 80 square feet (7.43 square meters), excluding vestibules, toilets, and closets. Room

arrangement should permit at least 2 feet 8 inches (81.28 centimeters) clearance at each side and at the foot of the examination table. A handwashing fixture and a counter or shelf space for writing shall be provided.

9.2.B2. Special-purpose examination rooms. Rooms for special clinics such as eye, ear, nose, and throat examinations, if provided, shall be designed and outfitted to accommodate procedures and equipment used. A handwashing fixture and a counter or shelf space for writing shall be provided.

9.2.B3. Treatment room(s). Rooms for minor surgical and cast procedures (if provided) shall have a minimum floor area of 120 square feet (11.15 square meters), excluding vestibule, toilet, and closets. The minimum room dimension shall be 10 feet (3.05 meters). A handwashing fixture and a counter or shelf for writing shall be provided.

9.2.B4. Observation room(s). Observation rooms for the isolation of suspect or disturbed patients shall have a minimum floor area of 80 square feet (7.43 square meters) and shall be convenient to a nurse or control station. This is to permit close observation of patients and to minimize possibilities of patients' hiding, escape, injury, or suicide. An examination room may be modified to accommodate this function. A toilet room with lavatory should be immediately accessible.

9.2.B5. Nurses station(s). A work counter, communication system, space for supplies, and provisions for charting shall be provided.

9.2.B6. Drug distribution station. This may be a part of the nurses station and shall include a work counter, sink, refrigerator, and locked storage for biologicals and drugs.

9.2.B7. Clean storage. A separate room or closet for storing clean and sterile supplies shall be provided. This storage shall be in addition to that of cabinets and shelves.

9.2.B8. Soiled holding. Provisions shall be made for separate collection, storage, and disposal of soiled materials.

9.2.B9. Sterilizing facilities. A system for sterilizing equipment and supplies shall be provided. Sterilizing procedures may be done on- or off-site, or disposables may be used to satisfy functional needs.

9.2.B10. Wheelchair storage space. Such storage shall be out of the direct line of traffic.

9.2.B11. The need for and number of required airborne infection isolation rooms in the rehabilitation facility shall be determined by an infection control risk assessment. When required, the airborne infection isolation room(s) shall comply with the general requirements of Section 7.2.C.

9.2.C. Radiology

Basic diagnostic procedures (these may be part of the outpatient service, off-site, shared, by contract, or by referral) shall be provided, including the following:

9.2.C1. Radiographic room(s). See Section 7.10 for special requirements.

9.2.C2. Film processing facilities.

9.2.C3. Viewing and administrative areas(s).

9.2.C4. Storage facilities for exposed film.

9.2.C5. Toilet rooms with handwashing facilities accessible to fluoroscopy room(s), if fluoroscopic procedures are part of the program.

9.2.C6. Dressing rooms or booths, as required by services provided, with convenient toilet access.

9.2.D. Laboratory

Facilities shall be provided within the outpatient department, or through an effective contract arrangement with a nearby hospital or laboratory service, for hematology, clinical chemistry, urinalysis, cytology, pathology, and bacteriology. If these services are provided on contract, the following laboratory facilities shall also be provided in (or be immediately accessible to) the outpatient facility:

9.2.D1. Laboratory work counter(s), with sink, vacuum, gas, and electric services.

9.2.D2. Lavatory(ies) or counter sink(s) equipped for handwashing.

9.2.D3. Storage cabinet(s) or closet(s).

9.2.D4. Specimen collection facilities with a water closet and lavatory. Blood collection facilities shall have seating space, a work counter, and handwashing facilities.

9.2.E. Housekeeping Room(s)

At least one housekeeping room per floor shall be provided. It shall contain a service sink and storage for housekeeping supplies and equipment.

9.2.F. Staff Facilities

Staff locker rooms and toilets shall be provided.

9.2.G. Engineering Service and Equipment Areas

The following shall be provided (these may be shared with other services provided capacity is appropriate for overall use):

9.2.G1. Equipment room(s) for boilers, mechanical equipment, and electrical equipment.

9.2.G2. Storage room(s) for supplies and equipment.

9.2.G3. Waste processing services:

a. Space and facilities shall be provided for the sanitary storage and disposal of waste.

b. If incinerators and/or trash chutes are used, they shall comply with NFPA 82.

c. Incinerators, if used, shall also conform to the standards prescribed by area air pollution regulations.

9.2.H. Details and Finishes

9.2.H1. Details shall comply with the following standards:

a. Minimum public corridor width shall be 5 feet (1.52 meters). Work corridors less than 6 feet (1.83 meters) long may be 4 feet (1.22 meters) wide.

b. Each building shall have at least two exits that are remote from each other. Other details relating to exits and fire safety shall comply with NFPA 101 and the standards outlined herein.

c. Items such as drinking fountains, telephone booths, vending machines, etc., shall not restrict corridor traffic or reduce the corridor width below the required minimum. Out-of-traffic storage space for portable equipment shall be provided.

d. The minimum door width for patient use shall be 2 feet 10 inches (86.36 centimeters). If the outpatient facility services hospital inpatients, the minimum width of doors to rooms used by hospital inpatients transported in beds shall be 3 feet 8 inches (1.12 meters).

e. Doors, sidelights, borrowed lights, and windows glazed to within 18 inches (46 centimeters) of the floor shall be constructed of safety glass, wired glass, or plastic glazing material that resists breakage and creates no dangerous cutting edges when broken. Similar materials shall be used in wall openings of playrooms and exercise rooms unless otherwise required for fire safety. Glazing materials used for shower doors and bath enclosures shall be safety glass or plastic.

f. Threshold and expansion joint covers shall be flush with the floor surface to facilitate use of wheelchairs and carts.

g. Handwashing facilities shall be located and arranged to permit proper use and operation. Particular care shall be taken to provide the required clearance for blade-type handle operation.

h. Provisions for hand drying shall be included at all handwashing facilities except scrub sinks.

i. Radiation protection for X-ray and gamma ray installations shall comply with Section 7.10.

j. The minimum ceiling height shall be 7 feet 10 inches (2.39 meters) with the following exceptions:

i. Boiler rooms shall have ceiling clearances not less than 2 feet 6 inches (76.20 centimeters) above the main boiler header and connecting piping.

ii. Radiographic and other rooms containing ceiling-mounted equipment shall have ceilings of sufficient height to accommodate the equipment and/or fixtures.

iii. Ceilings in corridors, storage rooms, toilet rooms, and other minor rooms shall not be less than 7 feet 8 inches (2.34 meters).

iv. Tracks, rails, and pipes suspended along the path of normal traffic shall be not less than 6 feet 8 inches (2.03 meters) above the floor.

k. Rooms containing heat-producing equipment (such as boiler or heater rooms) shall be insulated and ventilated to prevent occupied adjacent floor or wall surfaces from exceeding a temperature 10 degrees above the ambient room temperature.

9.2.H2. Finishes shall comply with the following standards:

a. Cubicle curtains and draperies shall be noncombustible or flame-retardant and shall pass both the large- and small-scale tests required by NFPA 701.

b. The flame-spread and smoke-developed ratings of finishes shall comply with Section 7.29 and Table 9. Where possible, the use of materials known to produce large amounts of noxious gases shall be avoided.

c. Floor materials shall be readily cleanable and appropriately wear-resistant. In all areas subject to wet cleaning, floor materials shall not be physically affected by liquid germicidal and cleaning solutions. Floors subject to traffic while wet, including showers and bath areas, shall have a nonslip surface.

d. Wall finishes shall be washable and, in the proximity of plumbing fixtures, shall be smooth and moisture resistant.

e. Wall bases in areas that are frequently subject to wet cleaning shall be monolithic and coved with the floor; tightly sealed to the wall; and constructed without voids.

f. Floor and wall areas penetrated by pipes, ducts, and conduits shall be tightly sealed to minimize entry of rodents and insects. Joints of structural elements shall be similarly sealed.

9.2.I. Design and Construction, Including Fire-Resistive Standards

9.2.I1. Construction and structural elements of freestanding outpatient facilities shall comply with recognized model building code requirements for offices and to the standards contained herein. Outpatient facilities that are an integral part of the hospital or that share common areas and functions shall comply with the construction standards for general hospitals. See applicable sections of this document for additional details.

9.2.I2. Interior finish materials shall have flame-spread and smoke-production limitations as described in NFPA 101. Wall finishes less than 4 mil thick applied over a noncombustible material are not subject to flame-spread rating requirements.

9.2.I3. Building insulation materials, unless sealed on all sides and edges, shall have a flame-spread rating of 25 or less and a smoke-developed rating of 150 or less when tested in accordance with NFPA 255.

9.2.J. Provision for Disasters
Seismic-force resistance of new construction for outpatient facilities shall comply with Section 1.4 and shall be given an importance factor of one. Where the outpatient facility is part of an existing building, that facility shall comply with applicable local codes. Special design provisions shall be made for buildings in regions that have sustained loss of life or damage to buildings from hurricanes, tornadoes, floods, or other natural disasters.

9.3 Primary Care Outpatient Centers

9.3.A. General
The primary care center provides comprehensive community outpatient medical services. The number and type of diagnostic, clinical, and administrative areas shall be sufficient to support the services and estimated patient load described in the program. All standards set forth in Sections 9.1 and 9.2 shall be met for primary care outpatient centers, with additions and modifications described herein. (See Section 9.4 for smaller care centers.)

9.3.B. Parking
Parking spaces for patients and family shall be provided at the rate of not less than two parking spaces for each examination and each treatment room. In addition, one space for each of the maximum number of staff persons on duty at any one shift will be provided. Adjustments, as described in Section 9.1.G, should be made where public parking, public transportation, etc., reduce the need for on-site parking.

9.3.C. Administrative Services

Each outpatient facility shall make provisions to support administrative activities, filing, and clerical work as appropriate. (See also Section 9.2.A.) Service areas shall include:

9.3.C1. Office(s), separate and enclosed, with provisions for privacy.

9.3.C2. Clerical space or rooms for typing and clerical work separated from public areas to ensure confidentiality.

9.3.C3. Filing cabinets and storage for the safe and secure storage of patient records with provisions for ready retrieval.

9.3.C4. Office supply storage (closets or cabinets) within or convenient to administrative services.

9.3.C5. A staff toilet and lounge in addition to and separate from public and patient facilities.

9.3.C6. Multiuse rooms for conferences, meetings, and health education. One room may be primarily for staff use but also available for public access as needed. In smaller facilities the room may also serve for consultation, etc.

9.3.D. Public Areas

Public areas shall be situated for convenient access and designed to promote prompt accommodation of patient needs, with consideration for personal dignity.

9.3.D1. Entrances shall be well marked and at grade level. Where entrance lobby and/or elevators are shared with other tenants, travel to the outpatient unit shall be direct and accessible to the disabled. Except for passage through common doors, lobbies, or elevator stations, patients shall not be required to go through other occupied areas or outpatient service areas. Entrance shall be convenient to parking and available via public transportation.

9.3.D2. A reception and information counter or desk shall be located to provide visual control of the entrance to the outpatient unit, and shall be immediately apparent from that entrance.

9.3.D3. The waiting area for patients and escorts shall be under staff control. The seating area shall contain not less than two spaces for each examination and/or treatment room. Where the outpatient unit has a formal pediatrics service, a separate, controlled area for pediatric patients shall be provided. Wheelchairs within the waiting area will be accommodated.

9.3.D4. Toilet(s) for public use shall be immediately accessible from the waiting area. In smaller units the toilet may be unisex and also serve for specimen collection.

9.3.D5. Drinking fountains shall be available for waiting patients. In shared facilities, drinking fountains may be outside the outpatient area if convenient for use.

9.3.D6. A control counter (may be part of the reception, information, and waiting room control) shall have access to patient files and records for scheduling of services.

9.3.E. Diagnostic

Provisions shall be made for X-ray and laboratory procedures as described in Sections 9.2.C and D. Services may be shared or provided by contract off-site. Each outpatient unit shall have appropriate facilities for storage and refrigeration of blood, urine, and other specimens. All standards set forth in Section 9.31 shall be met.

*9.3.F. Clinical Facilities

9.4 Small Primary (Neighborhood) Outpatient Facility

9.4.A. General

Facilities covered under this section are often contained within existing commercial or residential buildings as "store front" units, but they may also be a small, free-standing, new, or converted structure. The size of these units limits occupancy, thereby minimizing hazards and allowing for less stringent standards. Needed community services can therefore be provided at an affordable cost. The term *small structure* shall be defined as space and equipment serving four or fewer workers at any one time. Meeting all provisions of Section 9.2 for general outpatient facilities is desirable, but limited size and resources may preclude satisfying any but the basic minimums described. This section does not apply to outpatient facilities that are within a hospital, nor is it intended for the larger, more sophisticated units.

9.4.B. Location

The small neighborhood center is expected to be especially responsive to communities with limited income. It is essential that it be located for maximum accessibility and convenience. In densely populated areas, many of the patients might walk to services. Where a substantial number of patients rely on public transportation, facility location shall permit convenient access requiring a minimum of transfers.

9.4.C. Parking

Not less than one convenient parking space for each staff member on duty at any one time and not less than four spaces for patients shall be provided. Parking requirements may be satisfied with street parking, or by a nearby public parking lot or garage. Where the facility is within a shopping center or similar area, customer spaces may meet parking needs.

9.4.D. Administration and Public Areas

9.4.D1. Public areas shall include:

a. A reception and information center or desk.

b. Waiting space, including provisions for wheelchairs.

c. Patient toilet facilities.

9.4.D2. An office area for business transactions, records, and other administrative functions, separate from public and patient areas, shall be provided.

9.4.D3. General storage facilities for office supplies, equipment, sterile supplies, and pharmaceutical supplies shall be provided.

9.4.D4. Locked storage (cabinets or secure drawers) convenient to work stations shall be provided for staff valuables.

9.4.E. Clinical Facilities

9.4.E1. At least one examination room shall be available for each provider who may be on duty at any one time. Rooms may serve both as examination and treatment spaces (see Section 9.2.B1).

9.4.E2. A clean work area with a counter, a sink equipped for handwashing, and storage for clean supplies, shall be provided. This may be a separate room or an isolated area.

9.4.E3. A soiled holding room shall be provided (see Section 9.2.B8).

9.4.E4. Sterile equipment and supplies shall be provided to meet functional requirements. Sterile supplies may be prepackaged disposables or processed off-site.

9.4.E5. Locked storage for biologicals and drugs shall be provided.

9.4.E6. A toilet room containing a lavatory for handwashing shall be accessible from all examination and treatment rooms. Where a facility contains no more than three examination and/or treatment rooms, the patient toilet may also serve waiting areas.

9.4.F. Diagnostic Facilities

9.4.F1. The functional program shall describe where and how diagnostic services will be made available to the outpatient if these are not offered within the facility. When provided within the facility, these services shall meet the standards of Section 9.2.

9.4.F2. Laboratory services and/or facilities shall meet the following standards:

a. Urine collection rooms shall be equipped with a water closet and lavatory. Blood collection facilities shall have space for a chair and work counter. (The toilet room provided within the examination and treatment room may be used for specimen collection.)

b. Services shall be available within the facility or through a formal agreement or contract with a hospital or other laboratory for hematology, clinical chemistry, urinalysis, cytology, pathology, and bacteriology.

9.4.G. Details and Finishes
See Section 9.2.H.

9.4.H. Design and Construction

9.4.H1. Every building and every portion thereof shall be designed and constructed to sustain all dead and live loads in accordance with accepted engineering practices and standards. If existing buildings are converted for use, consideration shall be given to the structural requirements for concentrated floor loadings, including X-ray equipment, storage files, and similar heavy equipment that may be added.

9.4.H2. Construction and finishes may be of any type permitted for business occupancies as described in NFPA 101 and as specified herein.

9.4.I. Mechanical Standards
The following shall apply for the small outpatient facility of this section in lieu of Section 9.31:

9.4.I3. Heating and ventilation systems shall meet the following standards:

a. A minimum indoor winter-design-capacity temperature of 75°F (24°C) shall be set for all patient areas. Controls shall be provided for adjusting temperature as appropriate for patient activities and comfort.

b. All occupied areas shall be ventilated by natural or mechanical means.

c. Air-handling duct systems shall meet the requirements of NFPA 90A.

9.4.I4. Plumbing and other piping systems shall meet the following standards:

a. Systems shall comply with applicable codes, be free of leaks, and be designed to supply water at sufficient pressure to operate all fixtures and equipment during maximum demand.

b. Backflow preventer (vacuum breakers) shall be installed on all water supply outlets to which hoses or tubing can be attached.

c. Water temperature at lavatories shall not exceed 110°F (43°C).

d. All piping registering temperatures above 110°F (43°C) shall be covered with thermal insulation.

9.4.J. Electrical Standards
The following shall apply to the small outpatient facility of this section in lieu of Section 9.32:

9.4.J1. Prior to completion and acceptance of the facility, all electrical systems shall be tested and operated to demonstrate that installation and performance conform to applicable codes and functional needs.

9.4.J2. Lighting shall be provided in all facility spaces occupied by people, machinery, and/or equipment, and in outside entryways. An examination light shall be provided for each examination and treatment room.

9.4.J3. Sufficient duplex grounded-type receptacles shall be available for necessary task performance. Each examination and work table area shall be served by at least one duplex receptacle.

9.4.J4. X-ray equipment installations, when provided, shall conform to NFPA 70.

9.4.J5. Automatic emergency lighting shall be provided in every facility that has a total floor area of more than 1,000 square feet (92.9 square meters), and in every facility requiring stairway exit.

9.5 Outpatient Surgical Facility

9.5.A. General
Note: When invasive procedures are performed on persons who are known or suspected of having airborne infectious disease, these procedures should not be performed in the operating suite. These procedures shall be performed in a room meeting airborne infection isolation ventilation requirements or in a space using local exhaust ventilation. If the procedure must be performed in the operating suite, see the CDC's "Guidelines for Preventing the Transmission of Mycobacterium Tuberculosis in Health Care Facilities."

Outpatient surgery is performed without anticipation of overnight patient care. The functional program shall describe in detail staffing, patient types, hours of operation, function and space relationships, transfer provisions, and availability of offsite services.

If the outpatient surgical facility is part of an acute-care hospital or other medical facility, service may be shared to minimize duplication as appropriate. Where outpatient surgical services are provided within the same area or suite as inpatient surgery, additional space shall be provided as needed. If inpatient and outpatient procedures are performed in the same room(s), the functional program shall describe in detail scheduling and techniques used to separate inpatients and outpatients.

Visual and audible privacy should be provided by design and include the registration, preparation, examination, treatment, and recovery areas.

9.5.B. Size
The extent (number and types) of the diagnostic, clinical, and administrative facilities to be provided will be determined by the services contemplated and the estimated patient load as described in the narrative program. Provisions shall be made for patient examination, interview, preparation testing, and obtaining vital signs of patient for outpatient surgeries.

9.5.C. Parking
Four spaces for each room routinely used for surgical procedures plus one space for each staff member shall be provided. Additional parking spaces convenient to the entrance for pickup of patients after recovery shall be provided.

9.5.D. Administration and Public Areas
The following shall be provided:

9.5.D1. A covered entrance for pickup of patients after surgery.

9.5.D2. A lobby area including a waiting area, conveniently accessible wheelchair storage, a reception/information desk, accessible public toilets, public telephone(s), drinking fountain(s).

9.5.D3. Interview space(s) for private interviews relating to admission, credit, and demographic information gathering.

9.5.D4. General and individual office(s) for business transactions, records, and administrative and professional staff. These shall be separate from public and patient areas with provisions for confidentiality of records. Enclosed office spaces for administration and consultation shall be provided.

9.5.D5. Multipurpose or consultation room(s).

9.5.D6. A medical records room equipped for dictating, recording, and retrieval.

9.5.D7. Special storage, including locking drawers and/or cabinets, for staff personal effects.

9.5.D8. General storage facilities.

9.5.E. Sterilizing Facilities
A system for sterilizing equipment and supplies shall be provided. When sterilization is provided off site, adequate sterile supplies must be provided. If on-site processing facilities are provided, they shall include the following:

9.5.E1. Soiled Workroom

This room shall be physically separated from all other areas of the department. Work space should be provided to handle the cleaning and terminal sterilization/disinfection of all medical/surgical instruments and equipment. The soiled workroom shall contain work tables, sinks, flush-type devices, and washer/sterilizer decontaminators or other decontamination equipment. Pass-through doors and washer/sterilizer decontaminators should deliver into clean processing areas/workrooms.

9.5.E2. Clean Assembly/Workroom

This room should contain sterilization equipment. This workroom shall contain handwashing facilities, work space, and equipment for terminal sterilizing of medical and surgical equipment and supplies. Clean and soiled work areas should be physically separated. Access to sterilization room should be restricted.

This room is exclusively for the inspection, assembly, and packaging of medical/surgical supplies and equipment for sterilization. Area should contain work tables, counters, ultrasonic storage facilities for backup supplies and instrumentation, and a drying cabinet or equipment. The area should be spacious enough to hold sterilizer carts for loading or prepared supplies for sterilization.

9.5.E3. Clean/Sterile Supplies

Storage for packs, etc., shall include provisions for ventilation, humidity, and temperature control.

9.5.F. Clinical Facilities

Provisions should be made to separate pediatric from adult patients. This should include pre- and post-operative care areas and should allow for parental presence.

9.5.F1. At least one room shall be provided for examination and testing of patients prior to surgery, assuring both visual and audible privacy. This may be an examination room or treatment room as described in Sections 9.2.B1 and 3.

9.5.F2. Each operating room shall have a minimum clear area of 360 square feet (33.48 square meters), exclusive of cabinets and shelves, but may be larger to accommodate the functional plan which requires additional staff and/or equipment. Rooms that will be dedicated to laser procedure shall have a minimum clear area of 400 square feet (37.16 square meters), exclusive of cabinets and shelves. An emergency communication system connected with the surgical suite control station shall be provided. There shall be at least one X-ray film illuminator in each room. If the outpatient surgery service is to be integrated with hospital inpatient surgery service, at least one room shall be specifically designated for outpatient surgery. When the same operating rooms are used for inpatients, the functional program shall describe how scheduling conflicts will be avoided.

9.5.F3. Room(s) for post-anesthesia recovery of outpatient surgical patients shall be provided as required by volumes and procedure type. At least 3 feet (0.91 meter) shall be provided at each side and at the foot of each bed as needed for work and/or circulation. If pediatric surgery is part of the program, separation from the adult section and space for parents shall be provided. Soundproofing of the area and the ability to view the patient from the nursing station should be considered. Bedpans and bedpan-cleaning services shall be supplied in this area.

9.5.F4. A designated supervised recovery lounge shall be provided for patients who do not require post-anesthesia recovery but need additional time for their vital signs to stabilize before safely leaving the facility. This lounge shall contain a control station, space for family members, and provisions for privacy. It shall have convenient patient access to toilets large enough to accommodate a patient and an assistant. Handwashing and nourishment facilities must be included.

9.5.F5. The following services shall be provided in surgical service areas:

a. A control station located to permit visual surveillance of all traffic entering the operating suite.

b. A drug distribution station. Provisions shall be made for storage and preparation of medications administered to patients. A refrigerator for pharmaceuticals and double-locked storage for controlled substances shall be provided. Convenient access to handwashing facilities shall be provided.

c. Scrub facilities. Station(s) shall be provided near the entrance to each operating room and may service two operating rooms if needed. Scrub facilities shall be arranged to minimize incidental splatter on nearby personnel or supply carts.

d. Soiled workroom. The soiled workroom shall contain a clinical sink or equivalent flushing-type fixture, a work counter, a sink for handwashing, and waste receptacle(s).

e. Fluid waste disposal facilities. These shall be convenient to the general operating rooms. A clinical sink or equivalent equipment in a soiled workroom shall meet this standard.

f. Anesthesia storage facilities shall be in accordance with the standards detailed in Section 7.7.C9 for general hospitals.

g. Medical gas supply and storage with space for reserve nitrous oxide and oxygen cylinders.

h. Equipment storage room(s) for equipment and supplies used in the surgical suite.

i. Staff clothing change areas. Appropriate change areas shall be provided for staff working within the surgical suite. The areas shall contain lockers, showers, toilets, lavatories for handwashing, and space for donning scrub attire.

j. Outpatient surgery change areas. A separate area shall be provided for outpatients to change from street clothing into hospital gowns and to prepare for surgery. This area shall include waiting room(s), lockers, toilets, clothing change or gowning area(s), and space for administering medications. Provisions shall be made for securing patients' personal effects.

k. Stretcher storage area. This area shall be convenient for use and out of the direct line of traffic.

l. Lounge and toilet facilities for surgical staff. These shall be provided in facilities having three or more operating rooms. A toilet room will be provided near the recovery area.

m. Housekeeping room. Space containing a floor receptor or service sink and storage space for housekeeping supplies and equipment shall be provided exclusively for the surgical suite.

n. Space for temporary storage of wheelchairs.

o. Provisions for convenient access to and use of emergency crash carts at both the surgical and recovery areas.

9.5.G. Diagnostic Facilities
Diagnostic services shall be provided on- or off-site for preadmission tests as required by the functional program.

9.5.H. Details and Finishes
All details and finishes shall meet the standards in Section 9.2.H and below.

9.5.H1. Details shall conform to the following guidelines:

a. Minimum public corridor width shall be 6 feet (1.83 meters), except that corridors in the operating room section, where patients are transported on stretchers or beds, shall be 8 feet (2.44 meters) wide.

b. The separate facility or section shall comply with the "New Ambulatory Health Care Centers" section of NFPA 101 and as described herein. When the outpatient surgical unit is part of another facility that does not comply with, or exceeds, the fire safety requirements of NFPA 101, there shall be not less than one-hour separation between the outpatient surgical unit and other sections. The outpatient surgical facility shall have not less than two exits to the exterior. Exits, finishes, separation for hazardous areas, and smoke separation shall conform to NFPA 101.

c. Toilet rooms in surgery and recovery areas for patient use shall be equipped with doors and hardware that permit access from the outside in emergencies. When such rooms have only one opening or are small, the doors shall open outward or be otherwise designed to open without pressing against a patient who may have collapsed within the room.

d. Flammable anesthetics shall not be used in outpatient surgical facilities.

9.5.H2. Finishes shall conform to the following guidelines:

a. All ceilings and walls shall be cleanable. Those in sensitive areas such as surgical rooms shall be readily washable and free of crevices that can retain dirt particles. These sensitive areas shall have a finished ceiling that covers all overhead ductwork and piping. Finished ceilings may be omitted in mechanical and equipment spaces, shops, general storage areas, and similar spaces, unless required for fire-resistive purposes (see NFPA 99 and NFPA 70).

9.5.I. Plumbing
See Section 9.31.

9.5.J. Electrical
See Section 9.32.

9.5.K. Fire Alarm System
A manually operated, electrically supervised fire alarm system shall be installed in each facility as described in NFPA 101.

9.5.L. Mechanical
Heating, ventilation, and air conditioning shall be as described for similar areas in Section 9.31 and Table 2, except that the recovery lounge need not be considered a sensitive area and outpatient operating rooms may meet the standards for emergency trauma rooms. See Table 10 for filter efficiency standards.

9.6 Freestanding Emergency Facility

9.6.A. General
This section applies to the emergency facility that is separate from the acute-care hospital and that therefore requires special transportation planning to accommodate transfer of patients and essential services. The separate emergency facility provides expeditious emergency care where travel time to appropriate hospital units may be excessive. It may include provisions for temporary observation of patients until release or transfer.

Where hours of operation are limited, provisions shall be made in directional signs, notices, and designations to minimize potential for mistakes and loss of time by emergency patients seeking care during nonoperating hours.

Facility size, type, and design shall satisfy the functional program. In addition to standards in Sections 9.1 and 9.2, the following guidelines shall be met:

9.6.B. Location

The emergency facility shall be conveniently accessible to the population served and shall provide patient transfer to appropriate hospitals. In selecting location, consideration shall be given to factors affecting source and quantity of patient load, including highway systems, industrial plants, and recreational areas. Though most emergency patients will arrive by private cars, consideration should also be given to availability of public transportation.

9.6.C. Parking

Not less than one parking space for each staff member on duty at any one time and not less than two spaces for each examination and each treatment room shall be provided. Additional spaces shall be provided for emergency vehicles. Street, public, and shared lot spaces, if included as part of this standard, shall be exclusively for the use of the emergency facility. All required parking spaces shall be convenient to the emergency entrance.

9.6.D. Administrative and Public Areas

Administrative and public areas shall conform to the standards in Section 9.2.A with the following additions.

9.6.D1. Entrances shall be well marked, illuminated, and covered to permit protected transfer of patients from ambulance and/or automobiles. If a platform is provided for ambulance use, a ramp for wheelchairs and stretchers shall be provided in addition to steps. Door(s) to emergency services shall be not less than 4 feet (1.22 meters) wide to allow the passage of a stretcher and assistants. The emergency entrance shall have vision panels to minimize conflict between incoming and outgoing traffic and to allow for observation of the unloading area from the control station.

9.6.D2. Lobby and waiting areas shall satisfy the following requirements:

a. Convenient access to wheelchairs and stretchers shall be provided at the emergency entrance.

b. Reception and information function may be combined or separate. These areas shall provide direct visual control of the emergency entrance and access to the treatment area and the lobby. They shall include a public toilet with handwashing facilities, and a convenient telephone. Control stations will normally include triage function and shall be in direct communication with medical staff. Emergency entrance control functions shall include observation of arriving vehicles.

c. The emergency waiting area shall include provisions for wheelchairs and be separate from the area provided for scheduled outpatient service.

d. If so determined by the hospital infection control risk assessment, the diagnostic imaging waiting area may require special consideration to reduce the risk of airborne infection transmission. In these circumstances, public waiting areas shall be designed, ventilated, and maintained with available technologies such as enhanced general ventilation and air disinfection techniques similar to inpatient requirements for airborne infection isolation rooms. See the CDC's "Guidelines for Preventing the Transmission of Mycobacterium Tuberculosis in Health Care Facilities."

9.6.D3. Initial interviews may be conducted at the triage reception/control area. Facilities for conducting interviews on means of reimbursement, social services, and personal data shall include provisions for acoustical privacy. These facilities may be separate from the reception area but must be convenient to the emergency service waiting area.

9.6.D4. For standards concerning general and individual offices, see Section 9.2.A4.

9.6.D5. For standards concerning clerical space, see Section 9.2.A5.

9.6.D6. Multipurpose room(s) shall be provided for staff conferences. This room may also serve for consultation.

9.6.D7. For standards concerning special storage, see Section 9.2.A7.

9.6.D8. For standards concerning general storage, see Section 9.2.A8.

9.6.E. Clinical Facilities

See Section 9.2.B and, in addition, provide:

9.6.E1. A trauma/cardiac room for complex procedures as described in Section 9.5.F2 for the outpatient surgery unit. The trauma/cardiac room may be set up to accommodate more than one patient. Where the emergency trauma/cardiac room is set up for multipatient use, there shall be not less than 180 square feet (16.72 square meters) per patient area, and there shall be utilities and services for each patient. Provisions shall be included for patient privacy.

9.6.E2. In addition to wheelchair storage, a holding area for stretchers within the clinical area, away from traffic and under staff control.

9.6.E3. A poison control service with immediately accessible antidotes and a file of common poisons. Communication links with regional and/or national poison centers and regional EMS centers shall be provided. This service may be part of the nurses control and workstation.

9.6.E4. A nurses work and control station. This shall accommodate charting, files, and staff consultation activities. It shall be located to permit visual control of clinical area and its access. Communication links with the examination/treatment area, trauma/cardiac room, reception control, laboratory, radiology, and on-call staff shall be provided.

9.6.E5. A CPR emergency cart, away from traffic but immediately available to all areas including entrance and receiving areas.

9.6.E6. Scrub stations at each trauma/cardiac room. Water and soap controls shall not require use of hands.

9.6.E7. At least two examination rooms and one trauma/cardiac room (treatment room may also be utilized for examination).

9.6.F. Radiology
Standards stipulated in Section 9.2.C shall be met during all hours of operation. Radiographic equipment shall be adequate for any part of the body including, but not limited to, fractures. Separate dressing rooms are not required for unit(s) used only for emergency procedures.

9.6.G. Laboratory
See Section 9.2.D for applicable standards. In addition, immediate access to blood for transfusions and provisions for cross-match capabilities shall be provided.

9.6.H. Employee Facilities
See Section 9.2.F for applicable standards. In addition, facilities for on-call medical staff shall be provided.

9.6.I. Observation
Facilities shall be provided for holding emergency patients until they can be discharged or transferred to an appropriate hospital. Size, type, and equipment shall be as required for anticipated patient load and lengths of stay. One or more examination/treatment rooms may be utilized for this purpose. Each observation bed shall permit:

9.6.I1. Direct visual observation of each patient from the nurses station, except where examination/treatment rooms are used for patient holding. View from the duty station may be limited to the door.

9.6.I2. Patient privacy.

9.6.I3. Access to patient toilets.

9.6.I4. Secure storage of patients' valuables and clothing.

9.6.I5. Dispensing of medication.

9.6.I6. Bedpan storage and cleaning.

9.6.I7. Provision of nourishment (see Section 7.2.B15). In addition, meal provisions shall be made for patients held for more than four hours during daylight.

9.6.J. Mechanical
See Section 9.31 for applicable mechanical standards.

9.6.K. Plumbing
See Section 9.31 for applicable plumbing standards.

9.6.L. Electrical
See Section 9.32 for applicable electrical standards.

*9.7 Freestanding Birthing Center

The freestanding birthing center is "any health facility, place, or institution which is not a hospital and where births are planned to occur away from the mother's usual place of residence" (American Public Health Association, 1982).

All standards set forth in Sections 9.1 and 9.2 shall be met for new construction of birthing centers, with modifications described herein. Birthing rooms shall have available oxygen, vacuum, and medical air per Table 5, LDRP rooms.

9.7.A. Parking
Parking spaces for the client and family shall be provided at a rate of not less than two for each birth room. In addition, one space for each of the maximum number of staff persons on duty at any given time will be provided. Adjustments, as described in Section 9.1.G, should be made where public parking, public transportation, etc., reduce the need for on-site parking.

9.7.B. Administrative and Public Areas

9.7.B1. Entrance: The entrance to the birthing center shall be at ground level, well marked and illuminated. Provisions shall be made for emergency vehicle access.

9.7.B2. Provisions for the disabled: See Section 1.3.

9.7.B3. Public areas shall include:

a. A reception area with facility to accommodate outdoor wear.

b. A family room with a designated play area for children.

c. Child-proof electrical outlets.

d. A nourishment area for families to store and serve light refreshment of their dietary and cultural preferences shall include a sink and counter space, range, oven or microwave, refrigerator, cooking utensils, disposable tableware or dishwasher, storage space, and seating area.

e. Convenient access to toilet and handwashing facilities.

f. Convenient access to telephone service.

g. Convenient access to drinking fountain or potable drinking water with disposable cup dispenser.

9.7.B4. Staff area: A secure storage space for personal effects, toilet, shower, change and lounge area sufficient to accommodate staff needs shall be provided.

9.7.B5. Records: Space for performing administrative functions, charting, and secure record storage shall be provided.

9.7.B6. Drugs and biologicals: An area for locked storage for drugs and refrigeration for biologicals (separate from the nourishment area refrigerator) shall be provided.

9.7.B7. Clean storage: A separate area for storing clean and sterile supplies shall be provided.

9.7.B8. Soiled holding: Provisions shall be made for separate collection, storage, and disposal of soiled materials. Fluid waste may be disposed of in the toilet adjacent to the birth room.

9.7.B9. Sterilizing facilities: Sterile supplies may be prepackaged disposables or processed off-site. If instruments and supplies are sterilized on-site, an area for accommodation of sterilizing equipment appropriate to the volume of the birth center shall be provided.

9.7.B10. Laundry: May be done on- or off-site. If on-site, an area for laundry equipment with counter and storage space shelving shall be provided. Depending on size and occupancy of center, ordinary household laundry equipment may be provided. (Soiled laundry shall be held in the soiled holding area until deposited in the washer.)

9.7.C. Clinical Facilities
As needed, the following elements shall be provided for clinical services to satisfy the functional program.

9.7.C1. Birthing rooms: A minimum of two birthing rooms with storage space sufficient to accommodate belongings of occupants, bedding, equipment, and supplies needed for a family-centered childbirth shall be provided.

a. Birthing rooms shall be adequate in size to accommodate one patient, her family, and attending staff. A minimum floor area of 160 square feet (14.86 square meters) for new construction will be provided with a minimum dimension of 11 feet (3.35 meters). For renovation, a minimum floor area of 120 square feet (11.15 square meters) excluding vestibule, toilet, and closets will be provided with a minimum dimension of 10 feet (3.05 meters).

b. An area for equipment and supplies for routine and remedial newborn care, separate from the equipment supplies for maternal care, shall be provided in each birthing room in built-in cabinets, closets, or furniture.

c. Medicant, syringes, specimen containers, and instrument packs shall be contained in storage areas not accessible to children.

d. The plan for the birthing room shall be such that it will permit the need for emergency transfer by stretcher unimpeded.

9.7.C2. Toilet and bathing facilities: toilet, sink, and bath/shower facilities with appropriately placed grab bars shall be adjacent to each birthing room. Bath/shower facilities shall be shared by not more than two birthing rooms.

9.7.C3. Scrub areas: Handwashing fixtures with hands-free faucets shall be located conveniently accessible to the birthing rooms.

9.7.C4. Emergency equipment: An area for maternal and newborn emergency equipment and supplies (carts or trays) shall be designated out of the direct line of traffic and conveniently accessible to the birthing rooms.

9.7.C5. Communication: Each birthing room shall be equipped with a system for communicating to other parts of the center and to an outside telephone line.

9.8 Freestanding Outpatient Diagnostic and Treatment Facility

*9.8.A. General
This section applies to the outpatient diagnostic and treatment facility that is separate from the acute-care hospital. This facility is a new and emerging form of outpatient center which is capable of providing a wide array of outpatient diagnostic services and minimally invasive procedures.

The general standards for outpatient facilities set forth in Sections 9.1 and 9.2 shall be met for the freestanding outpatient diagnostic and treatment facility with two modifications.

9.8.A1. For those facilities performing diagnostic imaging and minimally invasive interventional procedures, all provisions of Section 7.10, General Hospital—Imaging Suite, shall also apply, except that adjacencies to emergency, surgery, cystoscopy, and outpatient clinics are not required.

9.8.A2. For those facilities performing nuclear medicine procedures, all provisions of Section 7.11, Nuclear Medicine, shall also apply, except that support services such as radiology, pathology, emergency room, and outpatient clinics are not required.

9.9 Endoscopy Suite

The endoscopy suite may be divided into three major functional areas: the procedure room(s), instrument processing room(s), and patient holding/preparation and recovery room or area. All standards set forth in Sections 9.31 and 9.32 shall be met for new construction of endoscopy suites with modifications described in Section 9.9.

Note: When invasive procedures are to be performed in this unit on persons who are known or suspected of having airborne infectious diseases, these procedures should not be performed in the operating suite. These procedures shall be performed in a room meeting airborne infection isolation ventilation requirements or in a space using local exhaust ventilation. If the procedure must be performed in the operating suite, see the CDC "Guidelines for Preventing the Transmission of Mycobacterium Tuberculosis in Health Care Facilities."

9.9.A. Procedure Room(s)

*9.9.A1. Each procedure room shall have a minimum clear area of 200 square feet (15.58 square meters) exclusive of fixed cabinets and built-in shelves.

9.9.A2. A freestanding handwashing fixture with hands-free controls shall be available in the suite.

9.9.A3. Station outlets for oxygen, vacuum (suction), and medical air. See Table 5.

9.9.A4. Floor covering shall be monolithic and joint free.

9.9.A5. A system for emergency communication shall be provided.

9.9.A6. Procedure rooms shall be designed for visual and acoustical privacy for the patient.

9.9.B. Instrument Processing Room(s)

9.9.B1. Dedicated processing room(s) for cleaning and disinfecting instrumentation must be provided. In an optimal situation, cleaning room(s) should be located between two procedure rooms. However, one processing room may serve multiple procedure rooms. Size of the cleaning room(s) is dictated by the amount of equipment to be processed.

Cleaning rooms should allow for flow of instrumentation from the contaminated area to the clean area, and finally, to storage. The clean equipment rooms, including storage, should protect the equipment from contamination.

9.9.B2. The decontamination room should be equipped with the following:

a. Two utility sinks remote from each other.

b. One freestanding handwashing fixture.

c. Work counter space(s).

d. Space and plumbing fixtures for automatic endoscope cleaners, sonic processor, and flash sterilizers (where required).

e. Ventilation system. Negative pressure shall be maintained and a minimum of 10 air changes per hour shall be maintained. A hood is recommended over the work counter. All air should be exhausted to the outside to avoid recirculation within the facility.

f. Outlets for vacuum and compressed air.

g. Floor covering shall be monolithic and joint free.

9.9.B3. Patient Holding/Prep/Recovery Area

The following elements should be provided in this area:

a. Each patient cubicle should be equipped with oxygen and suction outlets.

b. Cubicle curtains for patient privacy.

c. Medication preparation and storage with handwashing facilities.

d. Toilet facilities (may be accessible from patient holding or directly from procedure room(s) or both).

e. Change areas and storage for patients' personal effects.

f. Nurses reception and charting area with visualization of patients.

g. Clean utility room or area.

h. Janitor/housekeeping closet.

9.10 Cough-Inducing and Aerosol-Generating Procedures

All cough-inducing procedures performed on patients who may have infectious Mycobacterium tuberculosis shall be performed in rooms using local exhaust ventilation devices, e.g., booths or special enclosures with discharge HEPA filters or exhaust directly to the exterior. These procedures may also be performed in a room that meets the ventilation requirements for airborne infection isolation. See Table 2 for ventilation requirements.

9.11 Reserved

9.12 Reserved

9.13 Reserved

9.14 Reserved

9.15 Reserved

9.16 Reserved

9.17 Reserved

9.18 Reserved

9.19 Reserved

9.20 Reserved

9.21 Reserved

9.22 Reserved

9.23 Reserved

9.24 Reserved

9.25 Reserved

9.26 Reserved

9.27 Reserved

9.28 Reserved

9.29 Reserved

9.30 Special Systems

9.30.A. General

9.30.A1 Prior to acceptance of the facility, all special systems shall be tested and operated to demonstrate to the owner or his designated representative that the installation and performance of these systems conform to design intent. Test results shall be documented for maintenance files.

9.30.A2. Upon completion of the special systems equipment installation contract, the owner shall be furnished with a complete set of manufacturers' operating, maintenance, and preventive maintenance instructions, a parts lists, and complete procurement information including equipment numbers and descriptions. Operating staff persons shall also be provided with instructions for proper operation of systems and equipment. Required information shall include all safety or code ratings as needed.

9.30.A3. Insulation shall be provided surrounding special system equipment to conserve energy, protect personnel, and reduce noise.

9.30.B. Elevators

9.30.B1. Installation and testing of elevators shall comply with ANSI/ASME A17.1 for new construction and ANSI/ASME A17.3 for existing facilities. (See ASCE 7-93 for seismic design and control systems requirements for elevators.)

a. Cars shall have a minimum inside floor dimension of not less than 5 feet (1.52 meters).

b. Elevators shall be equipped with a two-way automatic level-maintaining device with an accuracy of ±½ inch (±1.27 centimeters).

c. Elevator call buttons and controls shall not be activated by heat or smoke. Light beams, if used for operating door reopening devices without touch, shall be used in combination with door-edge safety devices and shall be interconnected with a system of smoke detectors. This is so that the light control feature will be overridden or disengaged should it encounter smoke at any landing.

d. Elevator controls, alarm buttons, and telephones shall be accessible to wheelchair occupants and usable by the blind.

9.30.B2. Field inspections and tests shall be made and the owner shall be furnished with written certification stating that the installation meets the requirements set forth in this section as well as all applicable safety regulations and codes.

9.30.C. Waste Processing Services

9.30.C1. Storage and disposal. Facilities shall be provided for sanitary storage and treatment or disposal of waste using techniques acceptable to the appropriate health and environmental authorities. The functional program shall stipulate the categories and volumes of waste for disposal and shall stipulate the methods of disposal for each.

9.30.C2. Medical waste. Medical waste shall be disposed of either by incineration or other approved technologies. Incinerators or other major disposal equipment may be shared by two or more institutions.

a. Incinerators or other major disposal equipment may also be used to dispose of other medical waste where local regulations permit. Equipment shall be designed for the actual quantity and type of waste to be destroyed and should meet all applicable regulations.

b. Incinerators with 50-pounds-per-hour or greater capacities shall be in a separate room or outdoors; those with lesser capacities may be located in a separate area within the facility boiler room. Rooms and areas containing incinerators shall have adequate space and facilities for incinerator charging and cleaning, as well as necessary clearances for work and maintenance. Provisions shall be made for operation, temporary storage, and disposal of materials so that odors and fumes do not drift back into occupied areas. Existing approved incinerator installations, which are not in separate rooms or outdoors, may remain unchanged provided they meet the above criteria.

c. The design and construction of incinerators and trash chutes shall comply with NFPA 82.

*d. See Appendix A.

*e. See Appendix A.

9.30.C3. Nuclear Waste Disposal. See *Code of Federal Regulations,* title X, parts 20 and 35, concerning the handling and disposal of nuclear materials in health care facilities.

9.31 Mechanical Standards

Note: These requirements do not apply to small primary (neighborhood) outpatient facilities. See Section 9.4.I.

9.31.A. General

9.31.A1. The mechanical system should be designed for overall efficiency and life-cycle costing. Details for cost-effective implementation of design features are interrelated and too numerous (as well as too basic) to list individually. Recognized engineering procedures shall be followed for the most economical and effective results. A well-designed system can generally achieve energy efficiency at minimal additional cost and simultaneously provide improved patient comfort. Different geographic areas may have climatic and use conditions that favor one system over another in terms of overall cost and efficiency. In no case shall patient care or safety be sacrificed for conservation.

Mechanical, electrical, and HVAC equipment may be located either internally, externally, or in separate buildings.

9.31.A2. Remodeling and work in existing facilities may present special problems. As practicality and funding permit, existing insulation, weather stripping, etc., should be brought up to standard for maximum economy and efficiency. Consideration shall be given to additional work that may be needed to achieve this.

9.31.A3. Facility design consideration shall include site, building mass, orientation, configuration, fenestration, and other features relative to passive and active energy systems.

9.31.A4. Insofar as practical, the facility should include provisions for recovery of waste cooling and heating energy (ventilation, exhaust, water and steam discharge, cooling towers, incinerators, etc.).

9.31.A5. Facility design consideration shall include recognized energy-saving mechanisms such as variable-air-volume systems, load shedding, programmed controls for unoccupied periods (nights and weekends, etc.) and use of natural ventilation, site and climatic conditions permitting. Systems with excessive installation and/or maintenance costs that negate long-range energy savings should be avoided.

9.31.A6. Air-handling systems shall be designed with an economizer cycle where appropriate to use outside air. (Use of mechanically circulated outside air does not reduce need for filtration.)

It may be practical in many areas to reduce or shut down mechanical ventilation during appropriate climatic and patient-care conditions and to use open windows for ventilation.

9.31.A7. Mechanical equipment, ductwork, and piping shall be mounted on vibration isolators as required to prevent unacceptable structure-borne vibration.

9.31.A8. Supply and return mains and risers for cooling, heating, and steam systems shall be equipped with valves to isolate the various sections of each system. Each piece of equipment shall have valves at the supply and return ends.

9.31.A9. Upon completion of the equipment-installation contract, the owner shall be furnished with a complete set of manufacturers' operating, maintenance, and preventive maintenance instructions, a parts lists, and complete procurement information including equipment numbers and descriptions. Operating staff persons shall also be provided with instructions for properly operating systems and equipment. Required information shall include energy ratings as needed for future conservation calculations.

9.31.B. Thermal and Acoustical Insulation

9.31.B1. Insulation within the building shall be provided to conserve energy, protect personnel, prevent vapor condensation, and reduce noise.

9.31.B2. Insulation on cold surfaces shall include an exterior vapor barrier. (Material that will not absorb or transmit moisture will not require a separate vapor barrier.)

9.31.B3. Insulation, including finishes and adhesives on the exterior surfaces of ducts, piping, and equipment, shall have a flame-spread rating of 25 or less and a smoke-developed rating of 50 or less as determined by an independent testing laboratory in accordance with NFPA 255.

9.31.B4. If duct lining is used, it shall be coated and sealed, and shall meet ASTM C1071. These linings (including coatings, adhesives, and exterior surface insulation on pipes and ducts in spaces used as air supply plenums) shall have a flame-spread rating of 25 or less and a smoke-developed rating of 50 or less, as determined by an independent testing laboratory in accordance with NFPA 255. If existing lined ductwork is reworked in a renovation project, the liner seams and punctures shall be resealed.

9.31.B5. Duct linings exposed to air movement shall not be used in ducts serving operating rooms, delivery rooms, LDR rooms, and critical care units. This requirement shall not apply to mixing boxes and acoustical traps that have special coverings over such lining.

9.31.B6. Existing accessible insulation within areas of facilities to be modernized shall be inspected, repaired, and/or replaced, as appropriate.

9.31.B7. Duct lining shall not be installed within 15 feet (4.57 meters) downstream of humidifiers.

9.31.C. Steam and Hot Water Systems

9.31.C1. Boilers shall have the capacity, based upon the net ratings published by the Hydronics Institute or another acceptable national standard, to supply the normal heating, hot water, and steam requirements of all systems and equipment. Their number and arrangement shall accommodate facility needs despite the breakdown or routine maintenance of any one boiler. The capacity of the remaining boiler(s) shall be sufficient to provide hot water service for clinical, dietary, and patient use; steam for sterilization and dietary purposes; and heating for operating, delivery and birthing, labor, recovery, and intensive care. However, reserve capacity for facility space heating is not required in geographic areas where a design dry-bulb temperature of 25°F (–4°C) or more represents not less than 99 percent of the total hours in any one heating month as noted in ASHRAE's Handbook of Fundamentals, under the "Table for Climatic Conditions for the United States."

9.31.D. Air Conditioning, Heating, and Ventilation Systems

9.31.D1. All rooms and areas in the facility used for patient care shall have provisions for ventilation. The ventilation rates shown in Table 2 shall be used only as minimum standards; they do not preclude the use of higher, more appropriate rates. Though natural window ventilation for nonsensitive and patient areas may be employed, weather permitting, availability of mechanical ventilation should be considered for use in interior areas and during periods of temperature extremes. Fans serving exhaust systems shall be located at the discharge end and shall be readily serviceable. Air supply and exhaust in rooms for which no minimum total air change rate is noted may vary down to zero in response to room load. For rooms listed in Table 2, where VAV systems are used, minimum total air change shall be within limits noted. Temperature control shall also comply with these standards. To maintain asepsis control, airflow supply and exhaust should generally be controlled to ensure movement of air from "clean" to "less clean" areas, especially in critical areas. The ventilation systems shall be designed and balanced according to the requirements shown in Table 2 and in the applicable notes.

9.31.D2. General exhaust systems may be combined to enhance the efficiency of recovery devices required for energy conservation. Local exhaust systems shall be used whenever possible in place of dilution ventilation to reduce exposure to hazardous gases, vapors, fumes, or mists.

9.31.D3. Fresh air intakes shall be located at least 25 feet (7.62 meters) from exhaust outlets of ventilating systems, combustion equipment stacks, medical-surgical vacuum systems, plumbing vents, or areas that may collect vehicular exhaust or other noxious fumes. (Prevailing winds and/or proximity to other structures may require greater clearances.) Plumbing and vacuum vents that terminate at a level above the top of the air intake may be located as close as 10 feet (3.05 meters). The bottom of outdoor air intakes serving central systems shall be as high as practical, but at least 6 feet (1.83 meters) above ground level or, if installed above the roof, 3 feet (.91 meter) above roof level. Exhaust outlets from areas that may be contaminated shall be above roof level, arranged to minimize recirculation of exhaust air into the building, and directed away from personnel service areas.

9.31.D4. In new construction and major renovation work, air supply for operating and delivery rooms shall be from ceiling outlets near the center of the work area. Return air shall be near the floor level. Each operating and delivery room shall have at least two return-air inlets located as remotely from each other as practical. (Design should consider turbulence and other factors of air movement to minimize fall of particulates onto sterile surfaces.)

9.31.D5. Air supply for rooms used for invasive procedures shall be at or near the ceiling. Return or exhaust air inlets shall be near the floor level. Exhaust grills for anesthesia evacuation and other special applications shall be permitted to be installed in the ceiling.

*9.31.D6. Each space routinely used for administering inhalation anesthesia and inhalation analgesia shall be served by a scavenging system to vent waste gases. If a vacuum system is used, the gas-collecting system shall be arranged so that it does not disturb patients' respiratory systems. Gases from the scavenging system shall be exhausted directly to the outside. The anesthesia evacuation system may be combined with the room exhaust system, provided that the part used for anesthesia gas scavenging exhausts directly to the outside and is not part of the recirculation system. Scavenging systems are not required for areas where gases are used only occasionally, such as the emergency room, offices for routine dental work, etc. Acceptable concentrations of anesthetizing agents are unknown at this time. The absence of specific data makes it difficult to set specific standards. However, any scavenging system should be designed to reduce ambient concentrations of waste gases to safe levels. See Appendix A for additional information. It is assumed that anesthetizing equipment will be selected and maintained to minimize leakage and contamination of room air.

9.31.D7. The bottoms of ventilation (supply/return) openings shall be at least 3 inches (7.62 centimeters) above the floor.

9.31.D8. All central ventilation or air conditioning systems shall be equipped with filters with efficiencies equal to, or greater than, those specified in Table 10. Where two filter beds are required, filter bed no. 1 shall be located upstream of the air conditioning equipment and filter bed no. 2 shall be downstream of any fan or blowers. Filter efficiencies, tested in accordance with ASHRAE 52-92, shall be average. Filter frames shall be durable and proportioned to provide an airtight fit with the enclosing ductwork. All joints between filter segments and enclosing ductwork shall have gaskets or seals to provide a positive seal against air leakage. A manometer shall be installed across each filter bed having a required efficiency of 75 percent or more including hoods requiring HEPA filters.

*9.31.D9. If duct humidifiers are located upstream of the final filters, they shall be located at least 15 feet (4.57 meters) upstream of the final filters. Ductwork with duct-mounted humidifiers shall have a means of water removal. An adjustable high-limit humidistat shall be located downstream of the humidifier to reduce the potential of moisture condensing inside the duct. Humidifiers shall be connected to air flow proving switches that prevent humidification unless the required volume of air flow is present or high limit humidistats are provided. All duct takeoffs should be sufficiently downstream of the humidifier to ensure complete moisture absorption. Steam humidifiers shall be used. Reservoir-type water spray or evaporative pan humidifiers shall not be used.

9.31.D10. Air-handling duct systems shall be designed with accessibility for duct cleaning, and shall meet the requirements of NFPA 90A.

9.31.D11. Ducts that penetrate construction intended to protect against x-ray, magnetic, RFI, or other radiation shall not impair the effectiveness of the protection.

9.31.D12. Fire and smoke dampers shall be constructed, located, and installed in accordance with the requirements of NFPA 101, 90A, and the specific damper's listing requirements. Fans, dampers, and detectors shall be interconnected so that damper activation will not damage ducts. Maintenance access shall be provided at all dampers. All damper locations should be shown on design drawings. Dampers should be activated by fire or smoke sensors, not by fan cutoff alone. Switching systems for restarting fans may be installed for fire department use in venting smoke after a fire has been controlled. However, provisions should be made to avoid possible damage to the system due to closed dampers. When smoke partitions are required, heating, ventilation, and air conditioning zones shall be coordinated with compartmentation insofar as practical to minimize need to penetrate fire and smoke partitions.

9.31.D13. Hoods and safety cabinets may be used for normal exhaust of a space providing minimum air change rates are maintained. If air change standards in Table 2 do not provide sufficient air for proper operation of exhaust hoods and safety cabinets (when in use), makeup air (filtered and preheated) should be provided around these units to maintain the required airflow direction and exhaust velocity. Use of makeup air will avoid dependence upon infiltration from outdoor and/or from contaminated areas. Makeup systems for hoods shall be arranged to minimize "short circuiting" of air and to avoid reduction in air velocity at the point of contaminant capture.

9.31.D14. Laboratory hoods shall meet the following general standards:

a. Have an average face-velocity of at least 90–110 feet per minute (0.45–0.56 meters per second).

b. Be connected to an exhaust system to the outside which is separate from the building exhaust system.

c. Have an exhaust fan located at the discharge end of the system.

d. Have an exhaust duct system of noncombustible corrosion-resistant material as needed to meet the planned usage of the hood.

9.31.D15. Laboratory hoods shall meet the following special standards: In new construction and major renovation work, each hood used to process infectious or radioactive materials shall have a minimum face velocity of 90–110 feet per minute (0.45–0.56 meters per second) with suitable pressure-independent air modulating devices and alarms to alert staff of fan shutdown or loss of airflow. Each shall also have filters with a 99.97 percent efficiency (based on the dioctyl-phthalate [DOP] test method) in the exhaust stream, and be designed and equipped to permit the safe removal, disposal, and replacement of contaminated filters. Filters shall be as close to the hood as practical to minimize duct contamination. Fume hoods intended for use with radioactive isotopes shall be constructed of stainless steel or other material suitable for the particular exposure and shall comply with NFPA 801, *Facilities for Handling Radioactive Materials*. **Note:** Radioactive isotopes used for injections, etc., without probability of airborne particulates or gases may be processed in a clean-workbench-type hood where acceptable to the Nuclear Regulatory Commission.

9.31.D16. Exhaust hoods handling grease-laden vapors in food preparation centers shall comply with NFPA 96. All hoods over cooking ranges shall be equipped with grease filters, fire extinguishing systems, and heat-actuated fan controls. Cleanout openings shall be provided every 20 feet (6.10 meters) and at changes in direction in the horizontal exhaust duct systems serving these hoods. Each horizontal duct run shall have at least one cleanout opening. (Horizontal runs of ducts serving range hoods should be kept to a minimum.)

9.31.D17. The ventilation system for anesthesia storage rooms shall conform to the requirements of NFPA 99, including the gravity option. Mechanically operated air systems are optional in this room.

9.31.D18. The ventilation system for the space that houses ethylene oxide (ETO) sterilizers should be designed to:

a. Provide a dedicated (not connected to a return air or other exhaust system) exhaust system. Refer to 29 CFR Part 1910.1047.

b. All source areas shall be exhausted, including the sterilizer equipment room, service/aeration areas, over the sterilizer door, and the aerator. If the ETO cylinders are not located in a well-ventilated, unoccupied equipment space, an exhaust hood shall be provided over the cylinders. The relief valve shall be terminated in a well-ventilated, unoccupied equipment space, or outside the building. If the floor drain which the sterilizer(s) discharges to is not located in a well-ventilated, unoccupied equipment space, an exhaust drain cap shall be provided (coordinate with local codes).

c. Ensure that general airflow is away from sterilizer operator(s).

d. Provide a dedicated exhaust duct system for ETO. The exhaust outlet to the atmosphere should be at least 25 feet (7.62 meters) away from any air intake.

e. An audible and visual alarm shall activate in the sterilizer work area, and a 24-hour staffed location, upon loss of airflow in the exhaust system.

9.31.D19. Rooms with fuel-fired equipment shall be provided with sufficient outdoor air to maintain equipment combustion rates and to limit workstation temperatures.

9.31.D20. Gravity exhaust may be used, where conditions permit, for nonpatient areas such as boiler rooms, central storage, etc.

9.31.D21. The energy-saving potential of variable air volume systems is recognized and these standards herein are intended to maximize appropriate use of that system. Any system utilized for occupied areas shall include provisions to avoid air stagnation in interior spaces where thermostat demands are met by temperatures of surrounding areas.

*9.31.D22. Rooms or booths used for sputum induction, aerosolized pentamidine treatments, and other high-risk cough-inducing procedures shall be provided with local exhaust ventilation. See Appendix A for booth specifications.

9.31.D23. Non-central air handling systems, i.e., individual room units that are used for heating and cooling purposes (fan-coil units, heat pump units, etc.) shall be equipped with permanent (cleanable) or replaceable filters. The filters shall have a minimum efficiency of 68 percent weight arrestance. These units may be used as recirculating units only. All outdoor air requirements shall be met by a separate central air handling system with the proper filtration, as noted in Table 10.

9.31.E. Plumbing and Other Piping Systems

Unless otherwise specified herein, all plumbing systems shall be designed and installed in accordance with National Standard Plumbing Code.

9.31.E1. The following standards shall apply to plumbing fixtures:

a. The material used for plumbing fixtures shall be nonabsorptive and acid-resistant.

b. Water spouts used in lavatories and sinks shall have clearances adequate to avoid contaminating utensils and the contents of carafes, etc.

c. General handwashing facilities used by medical and nursing staff and all lavatories used by patients and food handlers shall be trimmed with valves that can be operated without hands. (Single lever or wrist blade devices may be used.) Blade handles used for this purpose shall not exceed 4½ inches (11.43 cm) in length. Handles on clinical sinks shall be at least 6 inches (15.24 cm) long. Freestanding scrub sinks and lavatories used for scrubbing in procedure rooms shall be trimmed with foot, knee, or ultrasonic controls (no single lever wrist blades).

d. Clinical sinks shall have an integral trap wherein the upper portion of the water trap provides a visible seal.

e. Showers and tubs shall have nonslip walking surfaces.

9.31.E2. The following standards shall apply to potable water supply systems:

a. Systems shall be designed to supply water at sufficient pressure to operate all fixtures and equipment during maximum demand. Supply capacity for hot- and cold-water piping shall be determined on the basis of fixture units, using recognized engineering standards. When the ratio of plumbing fixtures to occupants is proportionally more than required by the building occupancy and is in excess of 1,000 plumbing fixture units, a diversity factor is permitted.

b. Each water service main, branch main, riser, and branch to a group of fixtures shall have valves. Stop valves shall be provided for each fixture. Appropriate panels for access shall be provided at all valves where required.

c. Vacuum breakers shall be installed on hose bibbs and supply nozzles used for connection of hoses or tubing in laboratories, housekeeping sinks, bedpan-flushing attachments, and autopsy tables, etc.

d. Bedpan-flushing devices (may be cold water) shall be provided in each inpatient toilet room; however, installation is optional in psychiatric and alcohol-abuse units where patients are ambulatory.

e. Potable water storage vessels (hot and cold) not intended for constant use shall not be installed.

9.31.E3. The following standards shall apply to hot water systems:

a. The water-heating system shall have sufficient supply capacity at the temperatures and amounts indicated in Table 4. Water temperature is measured at the point of use or inlet to the equipment.

b. Hot-water distribution systems serving patient care areas shall be under constant recirculation to provide continuous hot water at each hot water outlet. The temperature of hot water for showers and bathing shall be appropriate for comfortable use but shall not exceed 110°F (43°C) (see Table 4).

9.31.E4. The following standards shall apply to drainage systems:

a. Drain lines from sinks used for acid waste disposal shall be made of acid-resistant material.

b. Drain lines serving some types of automatic blood-cell counters must be of carefully selected material that will eliminate potential for undesirable chemical reactions (and/or explosions) between sodium azide wastes and copper, lead, brass, and solder, etc.

c. Insofar as possible, drainage piping shall not be installed within the ceiling or exposed in operating and delivery rooms, nurseries, food preparation centers, food serving facilities, food storage areas, central services, electronic data processing areas, electric closets, and other sensitive areas. Where exposed, overhead drain piping in these areas is unavoidable, special provisions shall be made to protect the space below from leakage, condensation, or dust particles.

d. Floor drains shall not be installed in operating and delivery rooms.

*e. If a floor drain is installed in cystoscopy, it shall contain a nonsplash, horizontal-flow flushing bowl beneath the drain plate.

f. Drain systems for autopsy tables shall be designed to positively avoid splatter or overflow onto floors or back siphonage and for easy cleaning and trap flushing.

g. Building sewers shall discharge into community sewerage. When such a system is not available, the facility shall treat its sewage in accordance with local and state regulations.

h. Kitchen grease traps shall be located and arranged to permit easy access without the need to enter food preparation or storage areas. Grease traps shall be of capacity required and shall be accessible from outside of the building without need to interrupt any services.

i. Where plaster traps are used, provisions shall be made for appropriate access and cleaning.

j. In dietary areas, floor drains and/or floor sinks shall be of type that can be easily cleaned by removal of cover. Provide floor drains or floor sinks at all "wet" equipment (as ice machines) and as required for wet cleaning of floors. Provide removable stainless steel mesh in addition to grilled drain cover to prevent entry of large particles of waste which might cause stoppages. Location of floor drains and floor sinks shall be coordinated to avoid conditions where locations of equipment make removal of covers for cleaning difficult.

9.31.E5. The installation, testing, and certification of nonflammable medical gas and air systems shall comply with the requirements of NFPA 99. (See Table 5 for rooms requiring station outlets.)

9.31.E6. Clinical vacuum system installations shall be in accordance with NFPA 99. (See Table 5 for rooms which require station outlets.)

9.31.E7. All piping, except control-line tubing, shall be identified. All valves shall be tagged, and a valve schedule shall be provided to the facility owner for permanent record and reference.

9.31.E8. When the functional program includes hemodialysis, continuously circulated filtered cold water shall be provided.

9.31.E9. Provide condensate drains for cooling coils of type that may be cleaned as needed without disassembly. (Unless specifically required by local authorities, traps are not required for condensate drains.) Provide air gap where condensate drains empty into floor drains. Provide heater elements for condensate lines in freezer or other areas where freezing may be a problem.

9.31.E10. No plumbing lines may be exposed overhead or on walls where possible accumulation of dust or soil may create a cleaning problem or where leaks would create a potential for food contamination.

9.32 Electrical Standards

9.32.A. General

9.32.A1. All electrical material and equipment, including conductors, controls, and signaling devices shall be installed in compliance with applicable sections of NFPA 70 and NFPA 99 and shall be listed as complying with available standards of listing agencies, or other similar established standards where such standards are required.

9.32.A2. The electrical installations, including alarm and communication systems, shall be tested to demonstrate that equipment installation and operation is appropriate and functional. A written record of performance tests on special electrical systems and equipment shall show compliance with applicable codes and standards.

9.32.A3. Data processing and/or automated laboratory or diagnostic equipment, if provided, such equipment may require safeguards from power line disturbances.

9.32.B. Services and Switchboards

Main switchboards shall be located in an area separate from plumbing and mechanical equipment and shall be accessible to authorized persons only. Switchboards shall be convenient for use, readily accessible for maintenance, away from traffic lanes, and located in dry, ventilated spaces free of corrosive or explosive fumes, gases, or any flammable material. Overload protective devices shall operate properly in ambient room temperatures.

9.32.C. Panelboards

Panelboards serving normal lighting and appliance circuits shall be located on the same floor as the circuits they serve. Panelboards serving critical branch emergency circuits shall be located on each floor that has major users. Panelboards serving Life Safety emergency circuits may also serve floors above and/or below.

9.32.D. Lighting

9.32.D1. Lighting shall be engineered to the specific application.

9.32.D2. The Illuminating Engineering Society of North America (IES) has developed recommended lighting levels for health care facilities. The reader should refer to the *IES Handbook* (1993).

9.32.D3. Approaches to buildings and parking lots and all occupied spaces shall have fixtures for lighting that can be illuminated as necessary.

9.32.D4. Consideration should be given to the special needs for the elderly. Excessive contrast in lighting levels that make effective sight adaptation difficult should be minimized.

9.32.D5. A portable or fixed examination light shall be provided for examination, treatment, and trauma rooms.

9.32.E. Receptacles (Convenience Outlets)

Duplex grounded-type receptacles (convenience outlets) shall be installed in all areas in sufficient quantities for tasks to be performed as needed. Each examination and work table shall have access to a minimum of two duplex receptacles.

9.32.F. Equipment

9.32.F1. At inhalation anesthetizing locations, all electrical equipment and devices, receptacles, and wiring shall comply with applicable sections of NFPA 99 and NFPA 70.

9.32.F2. Fixed and mobile X-ray equipment installations shall conform to articles 517 and 660 of NFPA 70.

9.32.F3. Special equipment is identified in the following sections: Clinical Facilities, Radiology, and Laboratory. These sections shall be consulted to assure compatibility between programmatically defined equipment needs and appropriate power and other electrical connection needs.

9.32.G. Nurse Call System
Reserved.

9.32.H. Emergency Electrical Service
Emergency lighting and power shall be provided for in accordance with NFPA 99, NFPA 101, and NFPA 110.

9.32.I. Fire Alarm System
Any fire alarm system shall be as required by NFPA 101 and installed per NFPA 72.

9.32.J. Telecommunications and Information Systems

9.32.J1 Locations for terminating telecommunications and information system devices shall be provided.

9.32.J2. A space shall be provided for central equipment locations. Special air conditioning and voltage regulation shall be provided when recommended by the manufacturer.

Table 9

Flame-Spread and Smoke-Production Limitations on Interior Finishes

	Flame-spread rating	Smoke-production rating
Walls and ceiling		
Exitways, storage rooms, and areas of unusual fire hazard	25 or less (ASTM E84)	450 or less* (NFPA 258)
All other areas	75 or less (ASTM E84)	450 or less (NFPA 258)
Floors**		
Corridors and means of egress	Minimum of .45 watts/cm^2 (NFPA 253, Floor Radiant Panel Test)	

*Average of flaming and nonflaming values.

**See Section 1.3 for requirements relative to carpeting areas that may be subject to use by handicapped individuals. These areas include offices, waiting spaces, etc., as well as corridors that might be used by handicapped employees, visitors, or staff.

Table 10

Filter Efficiencies for Central Ventilation and Air Conditioning Systems in Outpatient Facilities

Area designation	No. filter beds	Filter bed no. 1	Filter bed no. 2
All areas for patient care, treatment, and/or diagnosis, and those areas providing direct service or clean supplies such as sterile and clean processing, etc.	2	30	90
Laboratories	1	80	—
Administrative, bulk storage, soiled holding areas, food preparation areas, and laundries	1	30	—

Notes: Additional roughing or prefilters should be considered to reduce maintenance required for main filters. The filtration efficiency ratings are based on dust spot efficiency per ASHRAE 52-76.

10. REHABILITATION FACILITIES

10.1 General Considerations

Rehabilitation facilities may be organized under hospitals (organized departments of rehabilitation), outpatient clinics, rehabilitation centers, and other facilities designed to serve either single- or multiple-disability categories including but not limited to: cerebrovascular, head trauma, spinal cord injury, amputees, complicated fractures, arthritis, neurological degeneration, genetic, and cardiac.

In general, rehabilitation facilities will have larger space requirements than general hospitals, have longer lengths of stay, and have less institutional and more residential environments.

10.1.A. Functional Units and Service Areas
Functional units and service areas shall include:

10.1.A1. Required units. Each rehabilitation facility shall contain a medical evaluation unit and one or more of the following units:

a. Psychological services unit.

b. Social services unit.

c. Vocational services.

10.1.A2. Required service areas. Each rehabilitation facility shall provide the following service areas, if they are not otherwise conveniently accessible to the facility and appropriate to program functions:

a. Patient dining, recreation, and day spaces.

b. Dietary unit.

c. Personal care facilities.

d. Unit for teaching activities of daily living.

e. Administration department.

f. Convenience store (i.e., expanded gift shop) with toiletries and other items accessible to patients during extended lengths of stay.

g. Engineering service and equipment areas.

h. Linen service.

i. Housekeeping rooms.

j. Employees' facilities.

k. Nursing unit.

10.1.A3. Optional units. The following special services areas, if required by the functional program, shall be provided as outlined in these sections. The sizes of the various departments will depend upon the requirements of the service to be provided:

a. Sterilizing facilities.

b. Physical therapy unit.

c. Occupational therapy unit.

d. Prosthetics and orthotics unit.

e. Speech and hearing unit.

f. Dental unit.

g. Radiology unit.

h. Pharmacy unit.

i. Laboratory facilities.

j. Home health service.

k. Outpatient services.

l. Therapeutic pool.

10.2 Evaluation Unit

10.2.A. Office(s) for Personnel

10.2.B. Examination Room(s)
Examination rooms shall have a minimum floor area of 140 square feet (13.01 square meters), excluding such spaces as the vestibule, toilet, closet, and work counter (whether fixed or movable). The minimum room dimension shall be 10 feet (3.05 meters). The room shall contain a lavatory or sink equipped for handwashing, a work counter, and storage facilities, and a desk, counter, or shelf space for writing.

10.2.C. Evaluation Room(s)
Evaluation room areas shall be arranged to permit appropriate evaluation of patient needs and progress and to determine specific programs of rehabilitation. Rooms shall include a desk and work area for the evaluators; writing and workspace for patients; and storage for supplies. Where the facility is small and workload light, evaluation may be done in the examination room(s).

10.2.D. Laboratory Facilities

Facilities shall be provided within the rehabilitation department or through contract arrangement with a nearby hospital or laboratory service for hematology, clinical chemistry, urinalysis, cytology, pathology, and bacteriology. If these facilities are provided through contract, the following minimum laboratory services shall be provided in the rehabilitation facility:

10.2.D1. Laboratory work counter(s) with a sink, and gas and electric service.

10.2.D2. Handwashing facilities.

10.2.D3. Storage cabinet(s) or closet(s).

10.2.D4. Specimen collection facilities. Urine collection rooms shall be equipped with a water closet and lavatory. Blood collection facilities shall have space for a chair and work counter.

10.2.E. Imaging Facilities

The following special services areas, if required by the functional program, shall be provided as outlined in Section 7.10.E. The sizes of the various departments will depend upon the requirements of the service to be provided:

10.2.E1. Electromyographic

10.2.E2. CAT Scan

10.2.E3. MRI

10.2.E4. Nuclear Medicine

10.2.E5. Radiographic

10.3 Psychological Services Unit

This shall include office(s) and work space for testing, evaluation, and counseling.

10.4 Social Services Unit

This shall include office space(s) for private interviewing and counseling.

10.5 Vocational Services Unit

Office(s) and work space for vocational training, counseling, and placement shall be provided.

10.6 Dining, Recreation, and Day Spaces

The following standards shall be met for patient dining, recreation, and day spaces (areas may be in separate or adjoining spaces):

10.6.A. Inpatients and Residents

A total of 55 square feet (5.11 square meters) per bed.

10.6.B. Outpatients

If dining is part of the day care program, a total of 55 square feet (5.11 square meters) per person shall be provided. If dining is not part of the program, at least 35 square feet (3.25 square meters) per person shall be provided for recreation and day spaces.

10.6.C. Storage

Storage spaces shall be provided for recreational equipment and supplies.

10.7 Dietary Department

10.7.A. General

Construction, equipment, and installation of food service facilities shall meet the requirements of the functional program. Services may consist of an on-site conventional food preparation system, a convenience food service system, or an appropriate combination thereof. On-site facilities should be provided for emergency food preparation and refrigeration.

The following facilities shall be provided as required to implement the food service selected:

10.7.A1. A control station for receiving food supplies.

10.7.A2. Food preparation facilities. Conventional food preparation systems require space and equipment for preparing, cooking, and baking. Convenience food service systems such as frozen prepared meals, bulk packaged entrees, individually packaged portions, and contractual commissary services require space and equipment for thawing, portioning, cooking, and/or baking.

10.7.A3. Handwashing facility(ies) located in the food preparation area.

10.7.A4. Patients' meal service facilities for tray assembly and distribution.

10.7.A5. Separate dining space shall be provided for staff.

10.7.A6. Warewashing space. This shall be located in a room or an alcove separate from food preparation and serving area. Commercial dishwashing equipment shall be provided. Space shall also be provided for receiving, scraping, sorting, and stacking soiled tableware and for transferring clean tableware to the using areas. A lavatory shall be conveniently available.

10.7.A7. Potwashing facilities.

10.7.A8. Storage areas for cans, carts, and mobile tray conveyors.

10.7.A9. Waste storage facilities. These shall be located in a separate room easily accessible to the outside for direct waste pickup or disposal.

10.7.A10. Office(s) or desk spaces for dietitian(s) or the dietary service manager.

10.7.A11. Toilets for dietary staff. Handwashing facilities shall be immediately available.

10.7.A12. Housekeeping room. This shall be located within the dietary department and shall contain a floor receptor or service sink and storage space for housekeeping equipment and supplies.

10.7.A13. Self-dispensing icemaking facilities. This may be in an area or room separate from the food preparation area but must be easily cleanable and convenient to dietary facilities.

10.8 Personal Care Unit for Inpatients

A separate room with appropriate fixtures and utilities shall be provided for patient grooming. The activities for daily living unit may serve this purpose.

10.9 Activities for Daily Living Unit

A unit for teaching daily living activities shall be provided. It shall include a bedroom, bath, kitchen, and space for training stairs. Equipment shall be functional. The bathroom must be an addition to other toilet and bathing requirements. The facilities should be similar to a residential environment so that the patient may learn to use them at home.

10.10 Administration and Public Areas

10.10.A. Entrance
A grade-level entrance, sheltered from the weather and able to accommodate wheelchairs, shall be provided.

10.10.B. Lobby
The lobby shall include:

10.10.B1. Wheelchair storage space(s).

10.10.B2. A reception and information counter or desk.

10.10.B3. Waiting space(s).

10.10.B4. Public toilet facilities.

10.10.B5. Public telephone(s).

10.10.B6. Drinking fountain(s).

10.10.B7. Convenience store (as described in Section 10.1.A2.f).

10.10.C. Interview Space(s)
Space for private interviews relating to social service, credit, and admissions shall be provided if not provided under Section 10.1.A1.

10.10.D. General or Individual Office(s)
General or individual offices for business transactions, records, and administrative and professional staffs shall be provided if not provided under Section 10.1.A2.

10.10.E. Multipurpose Room(s)
Multipurpose room(s) for conferences, meetings, health education, and library services shall be provided.

10.10.F. Storage of Patients' Personal Effects
Because their length of stay is longer than that of typical acute care patients, rehab patients may require more space for storage of personal effects.

10.10.G. General Storage
Separate space for office supplies, sterile supplies, pharmaceutical supplies, splints and other orthopedic supplies, and housekeeping supplies and equipment shall be provided.

10.11 Engineering Service and Equipment Areas

10.11.A. Equipment Rooms
Rooms for boilers, mechanical equipment, and electrical equipment shall be provided.

10.11.B. Storage Room(s)
Storage rooms for building maintenance supplies and yard equipment shall be provided.

10.11.C. Waste Processing Services

10.11.C1. Space and facilities shall be provided for the sanitary storage and disposal of waste.

10.11.C2. If provided, design and construction of incinerators and trash chutes shall be in accordance with NFPA 82 and shall also conform to the requirements prescribed by environmental regulations.

10.12 Linen Services

10.12.A. On-site Processing
If linen is to be processed on the site, the following shall be provided:

10.12.A1. Laundry processing room with commercial equipment that can process seven days' laundry within a regularly scheduled workweek. Handwashing facilities shall be provided.

10.12.A2. Soiled linen receiving, holding, and sorting room with handwashing and cart-washing facilities.

10.12.A3. Storage for laundry supplies.

10.12.A4. Clean linen storage, issuing, and holding room or area.

10.12.A5. Housekeeping room containing a floor receptor or service sink and storage space for housekeeping equipment and supplies.

10.12.B. Off-site Processing
If linen is processed off the rehabilitation facility site, the following shall be provided:

10.12.B1. Soiled linen holding room.

10.12.B2. Clean linen receiving, holding, inspection, and storage room(s).

10.13 Housekeeping Room(s)

In addition to the housekeeping rooms called for in certain departments, housekeeping rooms shall be provided throughout the facility as required to maintain a clean and sanitary environment. Each shall contain a floor receptor or service sink and storage space for housekeeping supplies and equipment.

10.14 Employee Facilities

In addition to the employee facilities such as locker rooms, lounges, toilets, or showers called for in certain departments, a sufficient number of such facilities to accommodate the needs of all personnel and volunteers shall be provided.

10.15 Nursing Unit (for Inpatients)

When inpatients are a part of the facility, each nursing unit shall provide the following:

10.15.A. Patient Rooms
Each patient room shall meet the following requirements:

10.15.A1. Maximum room occupancy shall be four patients. Larger units may be provided if justified by the functional program. At least two single-bed rooms with private toilet rooms shall be provided for each nursing unit.

10.15.A2. Minimum room areas exclusive of toilet rooms, closets, lockers, wardrobes, alcoves, or vestibules shall be 140 square feet (13.01 square meters) in single-bed rooms and 125 square feet (11.61 square meters) per bed in multi-bed rooms. In multi-bed rooms, a clearance of 3 feet 8 inches (1.12 meters) shall be maintained at the foot of each bed to permit the passage of equipment and beds.

10.15.A3. Each patient sleeping room shall have a window in accordance with Section 7.28.A11.

10.15.A4. A nurses' calling system shall be provided.

10.15.A5. Handwashing facilities shall be provided in each patient room.

10.15.A6. Each patient shall have access to a toilet room without having to enter the general corridor area. One toilet room shall serve no more than four beds and no more than two patient rooms. The toilet room shall contain a water closet and a handwashing fixture. The handwashing fixture may be omitted from a toilet room that serves single-bed and two-bed rooms if each such patient's room contains a handwashing fixture. Each toilet room shall be of sufficient size to ensure that wheelchair users will have access.

10.15.A7. Each patient shall have a wardrobe, closet, or locker with minimum clear dimensions of 1 foot 10 inches (55.88 centimeters) by 1 foot 8 inches (50.80 centimeters). An adjustable clothes rod and adjustable shelf shall be provided.

10.15.A8. Visual privacy shall be provided for each patient in multi-bed rooms.

10.15.B. Service Areas

The service areas noted below shall be in or readily available to each nursing unit. The size and disposition of each service area will depend upon the number and types of disabilities for which care will be provided. Although identifiable spaces are required for each indicated function, consideration will be given to alternative designs that accommodate some functions without designating specific areas or rooms. Such proposals shall be submitted for prior approval. Each service area may be arranged and located to serve more than one nursing unit, but at least one such service area shall be provided on each nursing floor. The following service areas shall be provided:

10.15.B1. Administrative center or nurse station.

10.15.B2. Nurses' office.

10.15.B3. Storage for administrative supplies.

10.15.B4. Handwashing facilities located near the nurse station and the drug distribution station. One lavatory may serve both areas.

10.15.B5. Charting facilities for nurses and doctors.

10.15.B6. Lounge and toilet room(s) for staff.

10.15.B7. Individual closets or compartments for safekeeping personal effects of nursing personnel, located convenient to the duty station or in a central location.

10.15.B8. Room for examination and treatment of patients. This room may be omitted if all patient rooms are single-bed rooms. It shall have a minimum floor area of 120 square feet (11.15 square meters), excluding space for vestibules, toilet, closets, and work counters (whether fixed or movable). The minimum room dimension shall be 10 feet (3.05 meters). The room shall contain a lavatory or sink equipped for handwashing, work counter, storage facilities, and a desk, counter, or shelf space for writing. The examination room in the evaluation unit may be used if it is conveniently located.

10.15.B9. Clean workroom or clean holding room.

10.15.B10. Soiled workroom or soiled holding room.

10.15.B11. Medication station. Provisions shall be made for convenient and prompt 24-hour distribution of medicine to patients. Distribution may be from a medicine preparation room, a self-contained medicine dispensing unit, or through another approved system. If used, a medicine preparation room shall be under the nursing staff's visual control and contain a work counter, refrigerator, and locked storage for biologicals and drugs. A medicine dispensing unit may be located at a nurse station, in the clean workroom, or in an alcove or other space under direct control of nursing or pharmacy staff.

10.15.B12. Clean linen storage. A separate closet or an area within the clean workroom shall be provided for this purpose. If a closed-cart system is used, storage may be in an alcove.

10.15.B13. Nourishment station. This shall be accessible to patients and contain a sink for handwashing, equipment for serving nourishment between scheduled meals, a refrigerator, storage cabinets, and icemaker-dispenser units to provide for patient service and treatment.

10.15.B14. Equipment storage room. This shall be for equipment such as I.V. stands, inhalators, air mattresses, and walkers.

10.15.B15. Parking for stretchers and wheelchairs. This shall be located out of the path of normal traffic.

10.15.B16. Multipurpose day room. Due to patients' length of stay, a day room shall be provided for patients to socialize on the unit.

10.15.C. Patient Bathing Facilities

Bathtubs or showers shall be provided at a ratio of one bathing facility for each eight beds not otherwise served by bathing facilities within patient rooms. At least one island-type bathtub shall be provided in each nursing unit. Each tub or shower shall be in an individual room or privacy enclosure that provides space for the private use of bathing fixtures, for drying and dressing, and for a wheelchair and an assistant. Showers in central bathing facilities shall be at least 4 feet (1.22 meters) square, curb-free, and designed for use by a wheelchair patient.

10.15.D. Patient Toilet Facilities

10.15.D1. A toilet room that does not require travel through the general corridor shall be accessible to each central bathing area.

10.15.D2. Doors to toilet rooms shall have a minimum width of 2 feet 10 inches (86.36 centimeters) to admit a wheelchair. The doors shall permit access from the outside in case of an emergency.

10.15.D3. A handwashing facility shall be provided for each water closet in each multi-fixture toilet room.

10.15.E.

The need for and number of required airborne infection isolation rooms in the rehabilitation facility shall be determined by an infection control risk assessment. When required, the airborne infection isolation room(s) shall comply with the general requirements of Section 7.2.C. These may be located within individual nursing units and used for normal acute care when not required for isolation cases, or they may be grouped as a separate isolation unit.

10.16 Sterilizing Facilities

When required by the functional program, a system for sterilizing equipment and supplies shall be provided.

10.17 Physical Therapy Unit

The following elements shall be provided:

10.17.A. Office Space

10.17.B. Waiting Space

10.17.C. Treatment Area(s)
For thermotherapy, diathermy, ultrasonics, hydrotherapy, etc., cubicle curtains around each individual treatment area shall be provided. Handwashing facility(ies) shall also be provided. One lavatory or sink may serve more than one cubicle. Facilities for collection of wet and soiled linen and other material shall be provided. As a minimum, one individual treatment area shall be enclosed within walls and have a door for access—minimum size 80 square feet (7.43 square meters). Curtained treatment areas shall have a minimum size of 70 square feet (6.51 square meters).

10.17.D. Exercise Area
Space requirements shall be designed to permit access to all equipment and be sized to accommodate equipment for physical therapy.

10.17.E. Storage for Clean Linen, Supplies, and Equipment

10.17.F. Patients' dressing areas, showers, lockers, and toilet rooms shall be provided as required by the functional program.

10.17.G. Wheelchair and Stretcher Storage
(Items 10.17.A, B, E, F, and G may be planned and arranged for shared use by occupational therapy patients and staff if the functional program reflects this sharing concept.)

10.18 Occupational Therapy Unit

The following elements shall be provided:

10.18.A. Office Space

10.18.B. Waiting Space

10.18.C. Activity Areas
Provisions shall be made for a sink or lavatory and for the collection of waste products prior to disposal.

10.18.D. Storage for Supplies and Equipment

10.18.E. Patients' dressing areas, showers, lockers, and toilet rooms shall be provided as required by the functional program.
(Items 10.18.A, B, D, and E may be planned and arranged for shared use by physical therapy patients and staff if the functional program reflects this sharing concept.)

10.19 Prosthetics and Orthotics Unit

The following elements shall be provided:

10.19.A. Work space for Technician(s)

10.19.B. Space for Evaluation and Fitting
This shall include provision for privacy.

10.19.C. Space for Equipment, Supplies, and Storage

10.20 Speech and Hearing Unit

This shall include:

10.20.A. Office(s) for Therapists

10.20.B. Space for Evaluation and Treatment

10.20.C. Space for Equipment and Storage

10.21 Dental Unit

The following elements shall be provided if required by the functional program:

10.21.A. Operatory
This shall contain a handwashing fixture.

10.21.B. Laboratory and Film Processing Facilities

10.22 Imaging Suite

This unit shall contain the following elements:

10.22.A.
Imaging room(s) shall be provided as required by the functional program. (See Section 7.10 for special requirements.)

10.23 Pharmacy Unit

The size and type of services to be provided in the pharmacy will depend upon the drug distribution system chosen and whether the facility proposes to provide, purchase, or share pharmacy services. This shall be explained in the narrative program. If a pharmacy is required by the functional program, provisions shall be made for the following functional areas:

10.23.A. Dispensing Area with a Handwashing Facility

10.23.B. Editing or Order Review Area

10.23.C. Area for Compounding

10.23.D. Administrative Areas

10.23.E. Storage Areas

10.23.F. Drug Information Area

10.23.G. Packaging Area

10.23.H. Quality-Control Area

10.24 Details and Finishes

Patients in a rehabilitation facility will be disabled to differing degrees. Therefore, high standards of safety for the occupants shall be provided to minimize accidents. All details and finishes for renovation projects as well as for new construction shall comply with the following requirements insofar as they affect patient services:

10.24.A. Details

10.24.A1. Compartmentation, exits, automatic extinguishing systems, and other details relating to fire prevention and fire protection in inpatient rehabilitation facilities shall comply with requirements listed in NFPA 101. In freestanding outpatient rehabilitation facilities, details relating to exits and fire safety shall comply with the appropriate business occupancy chapter of NFPA 101 and the requirements outlined herein.

10.24.A2. Items such as drinking fountains, telephone booths, vending machines, and portable equipment shall not restrict corridor traffic or reduce the corridor width below the required minimum.

10.24.A3. Rooms containing bathtubs, sitz baths, showers, and water closets subject to patient use shall be equipped with doors and hardware that will permit access from the outside in an emergency. When such rooms have only one opening or are small, the doors shall open outward or be otherwise designed to open without pressing against a patient who may have collapsed within the room.

10.24.A4. Minimum width of all doors to rooms needing access for beds shall be 3 feet 8 inches (1.12 meters). Doors to rooms requiring access for stretchers and doors to patient toilet rooms and other rooms needing access for wheelchairs shall have a minimum width of 2 feet 10 inches (86.36 centimeters). Where the functional program states that the sleeping facility will be for residential use (and therefore not subject to in-bed patient transport), patient room doors may be 3 feet (0.91 meter) wide, if approved by the local authority having jurisdiction.

10.24.A5. Doors between corridors and rooms or those leading into spaces subject to occupancy, except elevator doors, shall be swing-type. Openings to showers, baths, patient toilets, and other small, wet-type areas not subject to fire hazard are exempt from this requirement.

10.24.A6. Doors, except those to spaces such as small closets not subject to occupancy, shall not swing into corridors in a manner that obstructs traffic flow or reduces the required corridor width.

10.24.A7. Windows shall be designed to prevent accidental falls when open, or shall be provided with security screens where deemed necessary by the functional program.

10.24.A8. Windows and outer doors that may be frequently left open shall be provided with insect screens.

10.24.A9. Patient rooms intended for 24-hour occupancy shall have windows that operate without the use of tools and shall have sills not more than 3 feet (0.91 meter) above the floor.

10.24.A10. Doors, sidelights, borrowed lights, and windows glazed to within 18 inches (45.72 centimeters) of the floor shall be constructed of safety glass, wired glass, or plastic glazing material that resists breaking or creates no dangerous cutting edges when broken. Similar materials shall be used in wall openings of playrooms and exercise rooms. Safety glass or plastic glazing material shall be used for shower doors and bath enclosures.

10.24.A11. Linen and refuse chutes shall comply with NFPA 101.

10.24.A12. Thresholds and expansion joint covers shall be flush with the floor surface to facilitate use of wheelchairs and carts in new facilities.

10.24.A13. Grab bars shall be provided at all patient toilets, bathtubs, showers, and sitz baths. The bars shall have 1½ inches (3.81 centimeters) clearance to walls and shall be sufficiently anchored to sustain a concentrated load of 250 pounds (113.4 kilograms). Special consideration shall be given to shower curtain rods which may be momentarily used for support.

10.24.A14. Recessed soap dishes shall be provided in showers and bathrooms.

10.24.A15. Handrails shall be provided on both sides of corridors used by patients. A clear distance of 1½ inches (3.81 centimeters) shall be provided between the handrail and the wall, and the top of the rail shall be about 32 inches (81.28 centimeters) above the floor, except for special care areas such as those serving children.

10.24.A16. Ends of handrails and grab bars shall be constructed to prevent snagging the clothes of patients.

10.24.A17. Location and arrangement of handwashing facilities shall permit proper use and operation. Particular care should be given to clearance required for blade-type operating handles. Lavatories intended for use by disabled patients shall be installed to permit wheelchairs to slide under them.

10.24.A18. Mirrors shall be arranged for convenient use by wheelchair patients as well as by patients in a standing position.

10.24.A19. Provisions for hand drying shall be included at all handwashing facilities.

10.24.A20. Lavatories and handwashing facilities shall be securely anchored to withstand an applied vertical load of not less than 250 pounds (113.4 kilograms) on the front of the fixture.

10.24.A21. Radiation protection requirements of X-ray and gamma ray installations shall conform to necessary state and local laws. Provisions shall be made for testing the completed installation before use. All defects must be corrected before acceptance.

10.24.A22. The minimum ceiling height shall be 7 feet 10 inches (2.39 meters) with the following exceptions:

a. Boiler rooms shall have a ceiling clearance not less than 2 feet 6 inches (76.20 centimeters) above the main boiler header and connecting piping.

b. Ceilings of radiographic and other rooms containing ceiling-mounted equipment, including those with ceiling-mounted surgical light fixtures, shall have sufficient height to accommodate the equipment and/or fixtures.

c. Ceilings in corridors, storage rooms, toilet rooms, and other minor rooms may be not less than 7 feet 8 inches (2.34 meters).

d. Suspended tracks, rails, and pipes located in the path of normal traffic shall be not less than 6 feet 8 inches (2.03 meters) above the floor.

10.24.A23. Recreation rooms, exercise rooms, and similar spaces where impact noises may be generated shall not be located directly over patient bed areas unless special provisions are made to minimize such noise.

10.24.A24. Rooms containing heat-producing equipment (such as boiler or heater rooms and laundries) shall be insulated and ventilated to prevent any floor surface above from exceeding a temperature 10°F (6°C) above the ambient room temperature.

10.24.A25. Noise reduction criteria shown in Table 1 shall apply to partition, floor, and ceiling construction in patient areas.

10.24.B. Finishes

10.24.B1. Cubicle curtains and draperies shall be noncombustible or rendered flame retardant and shall pass both the large- and small-scale tests in NFPA 701.

10.24.B2. Floor materials shall be readily cleanable and appropriately wear-resistant for the location. Floor surfaces in patient areas shall be smooth, without irregular surfaces, to prevent tripping by patients using orthotic devices. Floors in food preparation or assembly areas shall be water-resistant. Joints in tile and similar material in such areas shall also be resistant to food acids. In all areas frequently subject to wet cleaning methods, floor materials shall not be physically affected by germicidal and cleaning solutions. Floors subject to traffic while wet, such as shower and bath areas, kitchens, and similar work areas, shall have a nonslip surface.

10.24.B3. Wall bases in kitchens, soiled workrooms, and other areas that are frequently subject to wet cleaning methods shall be monolithic and coved with the floor, tightly sealed within the wall, and constructed without voids that can harbor insects.

10.24.B4. Wall finishes shall be washable and, in the proximity of plumbing fixtures, shall be smooth and moisture-resistant. Finish, trim, and floor and wall construction in dietary and food preparation areas shall be free from spaces that can harbor pests.

10.24.B5. Floor and wall areas penetrated by pipes, ducts, and conduits shall be tightly sealed to minimize entry of pests. Joints of structural elements shall be similarly sealed.

10.24.B6. Ceilings throughout shall be readily cleanable. All overhead piping and ductwork in the dietary and food preparation area shall be concealed behind a finished ceiling. Finished ceilings may be omitted in mechanical and equipment spaces, shops, general storage areas, and similar spaces, unless required for fire-resistive purposes.

10.24.B7. Acoustical ceilings shall be provided for corridors in patient areas, nurse stations, day rooms, recreational rooms, dining areas, and waiting areas.

10.25 Design and Construction, Including Fire-Resistant Standards

10.25.A. Design
Except as noted below, construction of freestanding outpatient rehabilitation facilities shall adhere to recognized national model building codes and/or to NFPA 101 and the minimum requirements contained herein. Rehabilitation facilities that accommodate inpatients shall comply with the construction requirements for general hospitals as indicated in Section 7.

10.25.B. Interior Finishes
Interior finish materials for inpatient facilities shall comply with the flame-spread limitations and the smoke-production limitations set forth in NFPA 101.

10.25.C. Insulation Materials
Building insulation materials, unless sealed on all sides and edges, shall have a flame-spread rating of 25 or less and a smoke-developed rating of 150 or less when tested in accordance with NFPA 255-1984.

10.25.D. Provisions for Natural Disasters
For design and construction standards relating to hurricanes, tornadoes, and floods, see Section 7.29.F.

10.26 Reserved

10.27 Reserved

10.28 Reserved

10.29 Reserved

10.30 Special Systems

10.30.A. General

10.30.A1 Prior to acceptance of the facility, all special systems shall be tested and operated to demonstrate to the owner or his designated representative that the installation and performance of these systems conform to design intent. Test results shall be documented for maintenance files.

10.30.A2. Upon completion of the special systems equipment installation contract, the owner shall be furnished with a complete set of manufacturers' operating, maintenance, and preventive maintenance instructions, a parts lists, and complete procurement information including equipment numbers and descriptions. Operating staff persons shall also be provided with instructions for proper operation of systems and equipment. Required information shall include all safety or code ratings as needed.

10.30.A3. Insulation shall be provided surrounding special system equipment to conserve energy, protect personnel, and reduce noise.

10.30.B. Elevators

10.30.B1. All buildings having patient facilities (such as bedrooms, dining rooms, or recreation areas) or critical services (such as diagnostic or therapy) located on other than the main entrance floor shall have electric or hydraulic elevators. Installation and testing of elevators shall comply with ANSI/ASME A17.1, ANSI/ASME A17.3, or UFAS.

a. The number of elevators required shall be determined from a study of the facility plan and of the estimated vertical transportation requirements.

b. Hospital-type elevator cars shall have inside dimensions that accommodate a patient bed with attendants. Cars shall be at least 5 feet 8 inches (1.73 meters) wide by 9 feet (2.74 meters) deep. Car doors shall have a clear opening of not less than 4 feet (1.22 meters) wide and 7 feet (2.13 meters) high. In renovations, existing elevators that can accommodate patient beds used in the facility will not be required to be increased in size.

c. Elevator call buttons and controls shall not be activated by heat or smoke. Light beams, if used for operating door reopening devices without touch, shall be used in combination with door-edge safety devices and shall be interconnected with a system of smoke detectors. This is so that the light control feature will be overridden or disengaged should it encounter smoke at any landing.

10.30.B2. Field inspections and tests shall be made and the owner shall be furnished with written certification stating that the installation meets the requirements set forth in this section as well as all applicable safety regulations and codes.

10.30.C. Waste Processing Services

10.30.C1. Storage and disposal. Facilities shall be provided for sanitary storage and treatment or disposal of waste using techniques acceptable to the appropriate health and environmental authorities. The functional program shall stipulate the categories and volumes of waste for disposal and shall stipulate the methods of disposal for each.

10.30.C2. Medical waste. Medical waste shall be disposed of either by incineration or other approved technologies. Incinerators or other major disposal equipment may be shared by two or more institutions.

10.31 Mechanical Standards

10.31.A. General

10.31.A1. The mechanical system should be designed for overall efficiency and life cycle costing. Details for cost-effective implementation of design features are interrelated and too numerous (as well as too basic) to list individually. Recognized engineering procedures shall be followed for the most economical and effective results. A well-designed system can generally achieve energy efficiency at minimal additional cost and simultaneously provide improved patient comfort. Different geographic areas may have climatic and use conditions that favor one system over another in terms of overall cost and efficiency. In no case shall patient care or safety be sacrificed for conservation.

Mechanical, electrical, and HVAC equipment may be located either internally, externally, or in separate buildings.

10.31.A2. Remodeling and work in existing facilities may present special problems. As practicality and funding permit, existing insulation, weather stripping, etc., should be brought up to standard for maximum economy and efficiency. Consideration shall be given to additional work that may be needed to achieve this.

10.31.A3. Facility design consideration shall include site, building mass, orientation, configuration, fenestration, and other features relative to passive and active energy systems.

10.31.A4. Insofar as practical, the facility should include provisions for recovery of waste cooling and heating energy (ventilation, exhaust, water and steam discharge, cooling towers, incinerators, etc.).

10.31.A5. Facility design consideration shall include recognized energy-saving mechanisms such as variable-air-volume systems, load shedding, programmed controls for unoccupied periods (nights and weekends, etc.) and use of natural ventilation, site and climatic conditions permitting. Systems with excessive installation and/or maintenance costs that negate long-range energy savings should be avoided.

10.31.A6. Air-handling systems shall be designed with an economizer cycle when it is appropriate to use outside air. (Use of mechanically circulated outside air does not reduce the need for filtration.)

It may be practical in many areas to reduce or shut down mechanical ventilation during appropriate climatic and patient-care conditions and to use open windows for ventilation.

10.31.A7. Mechanical equipment, ductwork, and piping shall be mounted on vibration isolators as required to prevent unacceptable structure-borne vibration.

10.31.A8. Supply and return mains and risers for cooling, heating, and steam systems shall be equipped with valves to isolate the various sections of each system. Each piece of equipment shall have valves at the supply and return ends.

10.31.B. Thermal and Acoustical Insulation

10.31.B1. Insulation within the building shall be provided to conserve energy, protect personnel, prevent vapor condensation, and reduce noise.

10.31.B2. Insulation on cold surfaces shall include an exterior vapor barrier. (Material that will not absorb or transmit moisture will not require a separate vapor barrier.)

10.31.B3. Insulation, including finishes and adhesives on the exterior surfaces of ducts, piping, and equipment, shall have a flame-spread rating of 25 or less and a smoke-developed rating of 50 or less as determined by an independent testing laboratory in accordance with NFPA 255.

10.31.B4. If duct lining is used, it shall be coated and sealed and shall meet ASTM C1071. These linings (including coatings, adhesives, and exterior surface insulation on pipes and ducts in spaces used as air supply plenums) shall have a flame-spread rating of 25 or less and a smoke-developed rating of 50 or less, as determined by an independent testing laboratory in accordance with NFPA 255. If existing lined ductwork is reworked in a renovation project, the liner seams and punctures shall be resealed.

10.31.B5. Existing accessible insulation within areas of facilities to be modernized shall be inspected, repaired, and/or replaced, as appropriate.

10.31.B6. Duct lining shall not be installed within 15 feet (4.57 meters) downstream of humidifiers.

10.31.C. Steam and Hot Water Systems

10.31.C1. Boilers shall have the capacity, based upon the net ratings published by the Hydronics Institute or another acceptable national standard, to supply the normal heating, hot water, and steam requirements of all systems and equipment. Their number and arrangement shall accommodate facility needs despite the breakdown or routine maintenance of any one boiler. The capacity of the remaining boiler(s) shall be sufficient to provide hot water service for clinical, dietary, and patient use; steam for sterilization and dietary purposes; and heating for operating, recovery, and general patient rooms. However, reserve capacity for facility space heating is not required in geographic areas where a design dry-bulb temperature of 25°F (–4°C) or more represents not less than 99 percent of the total hours in any one heating month as noted in ASHRAE's *Handbook of Fundamentals*, under the "Table for Climatic Conditions for the United States."

10.31.C2. Boiler accessories including feed pumps, heat-circulating pumps, condensate return pumps, fuel oil pumps, and waste heat boilers shall be connected and installed to provide both normal and standby service.

10.31.D. Air Conditioning, Heating, and Ventilation Systems

10.31.D1. All rooms and areas in the facility used for patient care shall have provisions for ventilation. The ventilation rates shown in Table 2 shall be used only as minimum standards; they do not preclude the use of higher, more appropriate rates. Although natural window ventilation for nonsensitive areas and patient rooms may be employed, weather permitting, the availability of mechanical ventilation should be considered for use in interior areas and during periods of temperature extremes. Fans serving exhaust systems shall be located at the discharge end and shall be readily serviceable. Air supply and exhaust in rooms for which no minimum total air change rate is noted may vary down to zero in response to room load. For rooms listed in Table 2, where VAV systems are used, minimum total air change shall be within limits noted. Temperature control shall also comply with these standards. To maintain asepsis control, airflow supply and exhaust should generally be controlled to ensure movement of air from "clean" to "less clean" areas, especially in critical areas. The ventilation systems shall be designed and balanced according to the requirements shown in Table 2 and in the applicable notes.

10.31.D2. General exhaust systems may be combined to enhance the efficiency of recovery devices required for energy conservation. Local exhaust systems shall be used whenever possible in place of dilution ventilation to reduce exposure to hazardous gases, vapors, fumes, or mists.

10.31.D3. Fresh air intakes shall be located at least 25 feet (7.62 meters) from exhaust outlets of ventilating systems, combustion equipment stacks, medical-surgical vacuum systems, plumbing vents, or areas that may collect vehicular exhaust or other noxious fumes. (Prevailing winds and/or proximity to other structures may require greater clearances.) Plumbing and vacuum vents that terminate at a level above the top of the air intake may be located as close as 10 feet (3.05 meters). The bottom of outdoor air intakes serving central systems shall be as high as practical, but at least 6 feet (1.83 meters) above ground level, or, if installed above the roof, 3 feet (0.91 meters) above roof level. Exhaust outlets from areas that may be contaminated shall be above roof level, arranged to minimize recirculation of exhaust air into the building, and directed away from personnel service areas.

10.31.D4. All central ventilation or air conditioning systems shall be equipped with filters with efficiencies equal to, or greater than, those specified in Table 3. Where two filter beds are required, filter bed no. 1 shall be located upstream of the air conditioning equipment and filter bed no. 2 shall be downstream of any fan or blowers. Filter efficiencies, tested in accordance with ASHRAE 52-92, shall be average. Filter frames shall be durable and proportioned to provide an airtight fit with the enclosing duct work. All joints between filter segments and enclosing duct work shall have gaskets or seals to provide a positive seal against air leakage. A manometer shall be installed across each filter bed having a required efficiency of 75 percent or more including hoods requiring HEPA filters.

*10.31.D5. If duct humidifiers are located upstream of the final filters, they shall be located at least 15 feet (4.57 meters) upstream of the final filters. Ductwork with duct-mounted humidifiers shall have a means of water removal. An adjustable high-limit humidistat shall be located downstream of the humidifier to reduce the potential of condensation in the duct. All duct takeoffs should be sufficiently downstream of the humidifier to ensure complete moisture absorption. Steam humidifiers shall be used. Reservoir-type water spray or evaporative pan humidifiers shall not be used.

10.31.D6. Air-handling duct systems shall be designed with accessibility for duct cleaning and shall meet the requirements of NFPA 90A.

10.31.D7. Ducts that penetrate construction intended for X-ray or other ray protection shall not impair the effectiveness of the protection.

10.31.D8. Fire and smoke dampers shall be constructed, located, and installed in accordance with the requirements of NFPA 101, 90A, and the specific damper's listing requirements. Fans, dampers, and detectors shall be interconnected so that damper activation will not damage ducts. Maintenance access shall be provided at all dampers. All damper locations should be shown on design drawings. Dampers should be activated by fire or smoke sensors, not by fan cutoff alone. Switching systems for restarting fans may be installed for fire department use in venting smoke after a fire has been controlled. However, provisions should be made to avoid possible damage to the system due to closed dampers. When smoke partitions are required, heating, ventilation, and air conditioning zones shall be coordinated with compartmentation insofar as practical to minimize the need to penetrate fire and smoke partitions.

*10.31.D9. Hoods and safety cabinets may be used for normal exhaust of a space, provided that minimum air change rates are maintained. If air change standards in Table 2 do not provide sufficient air for proper operation of exhaust hoods and safety cabinets (when in use), makeup air (filtered and preheated) should be provided around these units to maintain the required airflow direction and exhaust velocity. Use of makeup air will avoid dependence upon infiltration from the outdoors and/or from contaminated areas. Makeup systems for hoods shall be arranged to minimize "short circuiting" of air and to avoid reduction in air velocity at the point of contaminant capture.

10.31.D10. Laboratory hoods shall meet the following general standards:

a. Have an average face-velocity of at least 75 feet per minute (0.38 meters per second).

b. Be connected to an exhaust system to the outside that is separate from the building exhaust system.

c. Have an exhaust fan located at the discharge end of the system.

d. Have an exhaust duct system of noncombustible corrosion-resistant material as needed to meet the planned usage of the hood.

10.31.D11. Laboratory hoods shall meet the following special standards:

a. Fume hoods, and their associated equipment in the air stream, intended for use with perchloric acid and other strong oxidants, shall be constructed of stainless steel or other material consistent with special exposures, and be provided with a water wash and drain system to permit periodic flushing of duct and hood. Electrical equipment intended for installation within such ducts shall be designed and constructed to resist penetration by water. Lubricants and seals shall not contain organic materials. When perchloric acid or other strong oxidants are only transferred from one container to another, standard laboratory fume hoods and the associated equipment may be used in lieu of stainless steel construction.

b. In new construction and major renovation work, each hood used to process infectious or radioactive materials shall have a minimum face velocity of 90–110 feet per minute (0.45–0.56 meters per second) with suitable pressure-independent air-modulating devices and alarms to alert staff of fan shutdown or loss of airflow. Each shall also have filters with a 99.97 percent efficiency (based on the dioctyl-phthalate [DOP] test method) in the exhaust stream and be designed and equipped to permit the safe removal, disposal, and replacement of contaminated filters. Filters shall be as close to the hood as practical to minimize duct contamination. Fume hoods intended for use with radioactive isotopes shall be constructed of stainless steel or other material suitable for the particular exposure and shall comply with NFPA 801, *Facilities for Handling Radioactive Materials*. **Note:** Radioactive isotopes used for injections, etc., without probability of airborne particulates or gases may be processed in a clean-workbench-type hood when acceptable to the Nuclear Regulatory Commission.

10.31.D12. Exhaust hoods handling grease-laden vapors in food preparation centers shall comply with NFPA 96. All hoods over cooking ranges shall be equipped with grease filters, fire extinguishing systems, and heat-actuated fan controls. Cleanout openings shall be provided every 20 feet (6.10 meters) and at changes in direction in the horizontal exhaust duct systems serving these hoods. (Horizontal runs of ducts serving range hoods should be kept to a minimum.)

10.31.D13. The ventilation system for the space that houses ethylene oxide (ETO) sterilizers should be designed to

a. Provide a dedicated (not connected to a return air or other exhaust system) exhaust system. Refer to 29 CFR Part 1910.1047.

b. Exhaust all source areas, including the sterilizer equipment room, service/aeration areas, over the sterilizer door, and the aerator. If the ETO cylinders are not located in a well-ventilated, unoccupied equipment space, an exhaust hood shall be provided over the cylinders. The relief valve shall be terminated in a well-ventilated, unoccupied equipment space or outside the building. If the floor drain that the sterilizer(s) discharges to is not located in a well-ventilated, unoccupied equipment space, an exhaust drain cap shall be provided (coordinate with local codes).

c. Ensure that general airflow is away from sterilizer operator(s).

d. Provide a dedicated exhaust duct system for ETO. The exhaust outlet to the atmosphere should be at least 25 feet (7.62 meters) away from any air intake.

e. Activate an audible and visual alarm in the sterilizer work area, and a 24-hour staffed location, upon loss of airflow in the exhaust system.

10.31.D14. Rooms with fuel-fired equipment shall be provided with sufficient outdoor air to maintain equipment combustion rates and to limit workstation temperatures.

10.31.D15. Gravity exhaust may be used, where conditions permit, for nonpatient areas such as boiler rooms, central storage, etc.

10.31.D16. The energy-saving potential of variable air volume systems is recognized, and these standards herein are intended to maximize appropriate use of that system. Any system utilized for occupied areas shall include provisions to avoid air stagnation in interior spaces where thermostat demands are met by temperatures of surrounding areas.

*10.31.D17. Rooms or booths used for sputum induction, aerosolized pentamidine treatments and other high-risk cough-inducing procedures shall be provided with local exhaust ventilation. See Appendix A for booth specifications.

10.31.D18. Non-central air handling systems, i.e., individual room units that are used for heating and cooling purposes (fan-coil units, heat pump units, etc.) shall be equipped with permanent (cleanable) or replaceable filters. The filters shall have a minimum efficiency of 68 percent weight arrestance. These units may be used as recirculating units only. All outdoor air requirements shall be met by a separate central air handling system with the proper filtration, as noted in Table 3.

10.31.E. Plumbing and Other Piping Systems.
Unless otherwise specified herein, all plumbing systems shall be designed and installed in accordance with *National Standard Plumbing Code,* chapter 14, Medical Care Facility Plumbing Equipment.

10.31.E1. The following standards shall apply to plumbing fixtures:

a. The material used for plumbing fixtures shall be non-absorptive and acid-resistant.

b. Waterspouts used in lavatories and sinks shall have clearances adequate to avoid contaminating utensils and the contents of carafes, etc.

c. General handwashing facilities used by medical and nursing staff and all lavatories used by patients and food handlers shall be trimmed with valves that can be operated without hands. (Single lever or wrist blade devices may be used.) Blade handles used for this purpose shall not exceed 4½ inches (11.43 cm) in length. Handles on clinical sinks shall be at least 6 inches (15.24 cm) long. Freestanding scrub sinks and lavatories used for scrubbing in procedure rooms shall be trimmed with foot, knee, or ultrasonic controls (no single lever wrist blades).

d. Clinical sinks shall have an integral trap wherein the upper portion of the water trap provides a visible seal.

e. Showers and tubs shall have nonslip walking surfaces.

10.31.E2. The following standards shall apply to potable water supply systems:

a. Systems shall be designed to supply water at sufficient pressure to operate all fixtures and equipment during maximum demand. Supply capacity for hot- and cold-water piping shall be determined on the basis of fixture units, using recognized engineering standards. When the ratio of plumbing fixtures to occupants is proportionally more than required by the building occupancy and is in excess of 1,000 plumbing fixture units, a diversity factor is permitted.

b. Each water service main, branch main, riser, and branch to a group of fixtures shall have valves. Stop valves shall be provided for each fixture. Appropriate panels for access shall be provided at all valves where required.

c. Vacuum breakers shall be installed on hose bibs and supply nozzles used for connection of hoses or tubing in laboratories, housekeeping sinks, bedpan-flushing attachments, and autopsy tables, etc.

d. Bedpan-flushing devices (may be cold water) shall be provided in each inpatient toilet room.

e. Potable water storage vessels (hot and cold) not intended for constant use shall not be installed.

10.31.E3. The following standards shall apply to hot water systems:

a. The water-heating system shall have sufficient supply capacity at the temperatures and amounts indicated in Table 4. Water temperature is measured at the point of use or inlet to the equipment.

b. Hot-water distribution systems serving patient care areas shall be under constant recirculation to provide continuous hot water at each hot water outlet. The temperature of hot water for showers and bathing shall be appropriate for comfortable use but shall not exceed 110°F (43°C) (see Table 4).

10.31.E4. The following standards shall apply to drainage systems:

a. Drain lines from sinks used for acid waste disposal shall be made of acid-resistant material.

b. Drain lines serving some types of automatic blood-cell counters must be of carefully selected material that will eliminate the potential for undesirable chemical reactions (and/or explosions) between sodium azide wastes and copper, lead, brass, and solder, etc.

c. Insofar as possible, drainage piping shall not be installed within the ceiling or exposed in operating rooms, food preparation centers, food serving facilities, food storage areas, central services, electronic data processing areas, electric closets, and other sensitive areas. Where exposed overhead drain piping in these areas is unavoidable, special provisions shall be made to protect the space below from leakage, condensation, or dust particles.

d. Floor drains shall not be installed in operating rooms.

e. If a floor drain is installed in cystoscopy, it shall contain a nonsplash, horizontal-flow flushing bowl beneath the drain plate.

f. Drain systems for autopsy tables shall be designed to positively avoid splatter or overflow onto floors or back siphonage and for easy cleaning and trap flushing.

g. Building sewers shall discharge into community sewerage. Where such a system is not available, the facility shall treat its sewage in accordance with local and state regulations.

h. Kitchen grease traps shall be located and arranged to permit easy access without the need to enter food preparation or storage areas. Grease traps shall be of capacity required and shall be accessible from outside the building without need to interrupt any services.

i. Where plaster traps are used, provisions shall be made for appropriate access and cleaning.

j. In dietary areas, floor drains and/or floor sinks shall be of a type that can be easily cleaned by removing the cover. Provide floor drains or floor sinks at all "wet" equipment (as ice machines) and as required for wet cleaning of floors. Provide removable stainless steel mesh in addition to a grilled drain cover to prevent entry of large particles of waste that might cause stoppages. Location of floor drains and floor sinks shall be coordinated to avoid conditions in which locations of equipment make removal of covers for cleaning difficult.

10.31.E5. The installation, testing, and certification of nonflammable medical gas and air systems shall comply with the requirements of NFPA 99. (See Table 5 for rooms requiring station outlets.)

10.31.E6. Clinical vacuum system installations shall be in accordance with NFPA 99. (See Table 5 for rooms that require station outlets.)

10.31.E7. All piping, except control-line tubing, shall be identified. All valves shall be tagged, and a valve schedule shall be provided to the facility owner for permanent record and reference.

10.31.E8. When the functional program includes hemodialysis, continuously circulated filtered cold water shall be provided.

10.31.E9. Provide condensate drains for cooling coils of a type that may be cleaned as needed without disassembly. (Unless specifically required by local authorities, traps are not required for condensate drains.) Provide an air gap where condensate drains empty into floor drains. Provide heater elements for condensate lines in freezers or other areas where freezing may be a problem.

10.31.E10. No plumbing lines may be exposed overhead or on walls where possible accumulation of dust or soil may create a cleaning problem or where leaks would create a potential for food contamination.

10.32. Electrical Standards

10.32.A. General

10.32.A1. All electrical material and equipment, including conductors, controls, and signaling devices shall be installed in compliance with applicable sections of NFPA 70 and NFPA 99 and shall be listed as complying with available standards of listing agencies or other similar established standards when such standards are required.

10.32.A2. The electrical installations, including alarm, nurse call, and communication systems shall be tested to demonstrate that equipment installation and operation is appropriate and functional. A written record of performance tests on special electrical systems and equipment shall show compliance with applicable codes and standards.

10.32.A3. Data processing and/or automated laboratory or diagnostic equipment, if provided, may require safeguards from power line disturbances.

10.32.B. Services and Switchboards

Main switchboards shall be located in an area separate from plumbing and mechanical equipment and shall be accessible to authorized persons only. Switchboards shall be convenient for use, readily accessible for maintenance, away from traffic lanes, and located in dry, ventilated spaces free of corrosive or explosive fumes, gases, or any flammable material. Overload protective devices shall operate properly in ambient room temperatures.

10.32.C. Panelboards

Panelboards serving normal lighting and appliance circuits shall be located on the same floor as the circuits they serve. Panelboards serving critical branch emergency circuits shall be located on each floor that has major users. Panelboards serving Life Safety emergency circuits may also serve floors above and/or below.

10.32.D. Lighting

10.32.D1. Lighting shall be engineered to the specific application.

10.32.D2. The Illuminating Engineering Society of North America (IES) has developed recommended lighting levels for health care facilities. The reader should refer to the *IES Handbook* (1993).

10.32.D3. Approaches to buildings and parking lots and all occupied spaces shall have fixtures for lighting that can be illuminated as necessary.

10.32.D4. Patient rooms shall have general lighting and night lighting. A reading light shall be provided for each patient. Reading light controls shall be readily accessible to patient(s). Incandescent and halogen light sources that produce heat should be avoided to prevent burns to the patient and/or bed linen. The light source should be covered by a diffuser or lens.

10.32.D5. Nursing unit corridors shall have general illumination with provisions for reducing light levels at night.

10.32.D6. Consideration should be given to the special needs of the elderly. Excessive contrast in lighting levels that makes effective sight adaptation difficult should be minimized.

10.32.E. Receptacles (Convenience Outlets)

10.32.E1. Each patient room shall have duplex-grounded receptacles. There shall be one at each side of the head of each bed and one on every other wall. Receptacles may be omitted from exterior walls where construction or room configuration makes installation impractical.

10.32.E2. Duplex-grounded receptacles for general use shall be installed approximately 50 feet (15.24 meters) apart in all corridors and within 25 feet (7.62 meters) of corridor ends.

10.32.E3. Electrical receptacle coverplates or electrical receptacles supplied from the emergency system shall be distinctively colored or marked for identification. If color is used for identification purposes, the same color should be used throughout the facility.

10.32.F. Equipment

10.32.F1. Ground-fault circuit interrupters (GFCIs) shall comply with NFPA 70. When GFCIs are used in critical areas, provisions shall be made to ensure that other essential equipment is not affected by activation of one interrupter.

10.32.F2. Fixed and mobile X-ray equipment installations shall conform to articles 517 and 660 of NFPA 70.

10.32.F3. Special equipment is identified in the following sections: Nursing Units, Support Areas, Rehabilitation Therapy, and Imaging, if applicable. These sections shall be consulted to ensure compatibility between programmatically defined equipment needs and appropriate power and other electrical connection needs.

10.32.G. Nurse Calling System

10.32.G1. A nurses calling system shall be provided. Each bed shall be provided with a call device. Two call devices serving adjacent beds may be served by one calling station. Calls shall activate a visible signal in the corridor at the patient's door or other appropriate location. In multicorridor nursing units, additional visible signals shall be installed at corridor intersections.

10.32.G2. A nurses emergency call shall be provided at each inpatient toilet, bath, sitz bath, and shower room. This emergency call shall be accessible to a collapsed patient lying on the floor. Inclusion of a pull cord will satisfy this standard. The emergency call shall be designed so that a signal activated at a patient's calling station will initiate a visible and audible signal distinct from the regular nurse calling system that can be turned off only at the patient calling station. The signal shall activate an annunciator panel at the nurses station or other appropriate location, a visible signal in the corridor at the patient's door, and at other areas defined by the functional program.

10.32.G3. Alternate technologies can be considered for emergency or nurse call systems. If radio frequency systems are utilized, consideration should be given to electromagnetic compatibility between internal and external sources.

10.32.H. Emergency Electrical Service

10.32.H1. As a minimum, nursing facilities or sections thereof shall have emergency electrical systems as required in NFPA 101, NFPA 110, and NFPA 99.

10.32.H2. When the nursing facility is a distinct part of an acute-care hospital, it may use the emergency generator system for required emergency lighting and power, if such sharing does not reduce hospital services. Such a shared system shall be designed with the capacity to meet the needs of both the hospital and rehabilitation facilities. Life support systems and their respective areas shall be subject to applicable standards of Section 7.32.

10.32.H3. An emergency electrical source shall provide lighting and/or power during an interruption of the normal electric supply.

10.32.I. Fire Alarm System
Fire alarm and detection systems shall be provided in compliance with NFPA 101 and NFPA 72.

10.32.J. Telecommunications and Information Systems

10.32.J1. Locations for terminating telecommunications and information system devices shall be provided.

10.32.J2. An area shall be provided for central equipment locations. Special air conditioning and voltage regulation shall be provided when recommended by the manufacturer.

11. PSYCHIATRIC HOSPITAL

11.1 General Conditions

11.1.A. Applicability
This section covers a psychiatric hospital intended for the care and treatment of inpatients and outpatients who do not require acute medical/surgical care services. See Section 7.6 for psychiatric units within acute care hospitals.

11.1.B. Functions
(See Section 1.1.F.)

11.1.C. Parking
In the absence of a formal parking study, the facility shall provide at least one space for each employee normally present during one weekday shift plus one space for every five beds or a total of 1.5 per patient. This ratio may be reduced when justified by availability of convenient public transportation and public parking. Additional parking may be required for outpatients or other services.

11.1.D. Swing Beds
Occupancy of a group of rooms within the facility may be changed to accommodate different patient groups based on age, sex, security level, or treatment programs.

11.1.E. Services
When the psychiatric facility is part of another facility, services such as dietary, storage, pharmacy, and laundry should be shared insofar as practical. In some cases, all ancillary service requirements will be met by the principal facility. In other cases, programmatic concerns and requirements may dictate separate services.

11.1.F. Environment
The facility should provide a therapeutic environment appropriate for the planned treatment programs. Security appropriate for the planned treatment programs shall be provided.

The unit should be characterized by a feeling of openness, with emphasis on natural light and exterior view. Interior finishes, lighting, and furnishings should suggest a residential rather than an institutional setting. These should, however, conform with applicable fire safety codes. Security and safety devices should not be presented in a manner to attract or challenge tampering by patients. Design, finishes, and furnishings should be such as will minimize the opportunity for residents to injure themselves or others. Special design considerations for injury and suicide prevention shall be given to the following elements:

- Visual control of nursing units and passive activity areas such as dayrooms and outdoor areas.

- Hidden alcoves or enclosed spaces.

- Areas secured from patients such as staff areas and mechanical space.

- Door closers, latch handles, and hinges.

- Door swings to private patient bathrooms.

- Shower, bath, toilet, and sink plumbing fixtures, hardware and accessories including grab bars and toilet paper holders.

- Windows, including interior and exterior glazing.

- Light fixtures, electrical outlets, electrical appliances, nurse call systems, and staff emergency assistance systems.

- Ceilings, ventilation grilles, and access panels in patient bedrooms and bathrooms.

- Sprinkler heads and other protrusions.

- Fire extinguisher cabinets and fire alarm pull stations.

11.2 General Psychiatric Nursing Unit

Each nursing unit shall include the following (see Section 1.2 for exceptions to standards when existing conditions make absolute compliance impractical).

11.2.A. Patient Rooms
Each patient room shall meet the following standards:

11.2.A1. Maximum room capacity shall be two patients.

11.2.A2. Patient room areas, exclusive of toilet rooms, closets, lockers, wardrobes, alcoves, or vestibules, shall be at least 100 square feet (9.29 square meters) for single-bed rooms and 80 square feet (7.43 square meters) per bed for multiple-bed rooms. Minor encroachments, including columns and lavatories, *that do not interfere with functions* may be ignored when determining space requirements for patient rooms. The areas noted herein are intended as recognized minimums and do not prohibit use of larger rooms when required for needs and functions.

Security rooms may be included if required by the treatment program. Security rooms shall be single-bed rooms designed to minimize potential for escape, hiding, injury to self or others, or suicide. Access to toilets, showers, and wardrobes shall be restricted. Security rooms may be centralized on one unit or decentralized among units.

11.2.A3. Windows or vents in psychiatric units shall be arranged and located so that they can be opened from the inside to permit venting of combustion products and to permit any occupant direct access to fresh air in emergencies. The operation of operable windows shall be restricted. When windows or vents require the use of tools or keys for operation, the tools or keys shall be located on the same floor in a prominent location accessible to staff. Windows in buildings designed with approved, engineered smoke-control systems may be of fixed construction. Security glazing and/or other appropriate security features shall be used at all windows of the nursing unit and other patient activity and treatment areas to reduce the possibility of patient injury or escape.

11.2.A4. Each patient shall have access to a toilet room without having to enter the general corridor area.

(This direct access requirement may be disregarded if it conflicts with the supervision of patients as required by the treatment program.)

One toilet room shall serve no more than four beds and no more than two patient rooms. The toilet room shall contain a water closet and a handwashing fixture, and the door should swing outward or be double acting.

11.2.A5. Each patient shall have within his or her room a separate wardrobe, locker, or closet suitable for hanging full-length garments and for storing personal effects. Adequate storage should be available for a daily change of clothes for seven days. When the treatment program indicates, shelves for folded garments may be used instead of hanging garments.

11.2.A6. There shall be a desk or writing surface in each room for patient use.

11.2.B. Service Areas
Provisions for the services noted below shall be located in or be readily available to each nursing unit. Each service area may be arranged and located to serve more than one nursing unit but, unless noted otherwise, at least one such service area shall be provided on each nursing floor. Where the words *room* or *office* are used, a separate, enclosed space for the one named function is intended; otherwise, the described area may be a specific space in another room or common area.

11.2.B1. Administrative center or nurse station.

11.2.B2. Office(s) for staff.

11.2.B3. Administrative supplies storage.

11.2.B4. Handwashing fixtures (see Section 7.2.B4).

11.2.B5. A separate charting area shall be provided with provisions for acoustical and patient file privacy.

11.2.B6. Toilet room(s) for staff.

11.2.B7. Staff lounge facilities.

11.2.B8. Securable closets or cabinet compartments for the personal effects of nursing personnel, conveniently located to the duty station. At a minimum, these shall be large enough for purses and billfolds.

11.2.B9. Clean workroom or clean holding room (see Section 7.2.B11).

11.2.B10. Soiled workroom (see Section 7.2.B12).

11.2.B11. Drug distribution station (see Section 7.2.B13).

11.2.B12. Clean linen storage (see Section 7.2.B14).

11.2.B13. Food service within the unit may be one or a combination of the following:

a. A nourishment station.

b. A kitchenette designed for patient use with staff control of heating and cooking devices.

c. A kitchen service within the unit, including a sink equipped for handwashing, storage space, refrigerator, and facilities for meal preparation.

11.2.B14. Ice machine (see Section 7.2.B16).

11.2.B15. A bathtub or shower shall be provided for each six beds not otherwise served by bathing facilities within the patient rooms. Bathing facilities should be designed and located for patient convenience and privacy.

11.2.B16. At least two separate social spaces, one appropriate for noisy activities and one for quiet activities, shall be provided. The combined area shall be at least 25 square feet (2.32 square meters) per patient with at least 120 square feet (11.15 square meters) for each of the two spaces. This space may be shared by dining activities if an additional 15 square feet (1.39 square meters) per patient is added; otherwise, provide 20 square feet (1.86 square meters) per patient for dining. Dining facilities may be located off the nursing unit in a central area.

11.2.B17. Space for group therapy shall be provided. This may be combined with the quiet space noted above when the unit accommodates not more than 12 patients and when at least 225 square feet (20.92 square meters) of enclosed private space is available for group therapy activities.

11.2.B18. Patient laundry facilities with an automatic washer and dryer shall be provided.

11.2.B19. A secured storage area for patients' effects determined potentially harmful (razors, nail files, cigarette lighters, etc.). This area will be controlled by staff.

The following elements shall also be provided, but may be either within the psychiatric unit or immediately accessible to it unless otherwise dictated by the program:

11.2.B20. Equipment storage room.

11.2.B21. Storage space for wheelchairs may be outside the psychiatric unit, provided that provisions are made for convenient access as needed for disabled patients.

11.2.B22. Examination and treatment room(s). The examination and treatment room(s) may serve several nursing units and may be on a different floor if conveniently located for routine use. Examination rooms shall have a minimum floor area of 120 square feet (11.15 square meters) excluding space for vestibule, toilets, and closets. The room shall contain a lavatory or sink equipped for handwashing; storage facilities; and a desk, counter, or shelf space for writing.

11.2.B23. Emergency equipment storage. Space shall be provided for emergency equipment that is under direct control of the nursing staff, such as a CPR cart. This space shall be in close proximity to a nurse station; it may serve more than one unit.

11.2.B24. Housekeeping room (see Section 7.2.B22).

11.2.B25. A visitor room for patients to meet with friends or family with a minimum floor space of 100 square feet (9.29 square meters).

11.2.B26. A quiet room for a patient who needs to be alone for a short period of time but does not require a seclusion room. A minimum of 80 square feet (7.43 square meters) is required. The visitor room may serve this purpose.

11.2.B27. Separate consultation room(s) with minimum floor space of 100 square feet (9.29 square meters) each provided at a room-to-bed ratio of one consultation room for each 12 psychiatric beds. The room(s) shall be designed for acoustical and visual privacy and constructed to achieve a level of voice privacy of 50 STC (which in terms of vocal privacy means that some loud or raised speech is heard only by straining, but is not intelligible). The visitor room may serve as a consultation room.

11.2.B28. A conference and treatment planning room for use by the psychiatric unit. This room may be combined with the charting room.

11.2.C. Seclusion Treatment Room

There shall be at least one seclusion room for up to 24 beds or a major fraction thereof. The seclusion treatment room is intended for short-term occupancy by violent or suicidal patients. Within the psychiatric nursing unit, this space provides for patients requiring security and protection. The room(s) shall be located for direct nursing staff supervision. Each room shall be for only one patient. It shall have an area of at least 60 square feet (5.58quare meters) and shall be constructed to prevent patient hiding, escape, injury, or suicide. When restraint beds are required by the functional program, 80 square feet (7.43 square meters) shall be required. If a facility has more than one psychiatric nursing unit, the number of seclusion rooms shall be a function of the total number of psychiatric beds in the facility. Seclusion rooms may be grouped together. Special fixtures and hardware for electrical circuits shall be used. Doors shall be 3 feet 8 inches (1.12 meters) wide and shall permit staff observation of the patient while also maintaining provisions for patient privacy. Minimum ceiling height shall be 9 feet (2.74 meters). Seclusion treatment rooms shall be accessed by an anteroom or vestibule that also provides direct access to a toilet room. The toilet room and anteroom shall be large enough to safely manage the patient. The seclusion room door shall swing out.

When the interior of the seclusion treatment room is padded with combustible materials, these materials shall be of a type acceptable to the local authority having jurisdiction. The room area, including floor, walls, ceilings, and all openings shall be protected with not less than one-hour-rated construction.

11.2.D.

The need for and number of required airborne infection isolation rooms in the psychiatric hospital shall be determined by an infection control risk assessment. When required, the airborne infection isolation room(s) shall comply with the general requirements of Section 7.2.C.

11.3 Child Psychiatric Unit

The standards of Section 11.2 shall be applied to child units with the following exceptions.

11.3.A. Patient Rooms

11.3.A1. Maximum room capacity shall be four children.

11.3.A2. Patient room areas (with beds or cribs) shall be 100 square feet (9.29 square meters) for single bedrooms; 80 square feet (7.43 square meters) per bed and 60 square feet (5.58 square meters) per crib in multiple-bed rooms.

11.3.A3. Storage space shall be provided for toys, equipment, extra cribs and beds, and cots or recliners for parents who might stay overnight.

11.3.B. Service Areas

11.3.B1. The combined area for social activities shall be 35 square feet (3.25 square meters) per patient.

11.4 Geriatric, Alzheimer's, and Other Dementia Unit

The standards of Section 11.2 shall be applied to geriatric units with the following exceptions.

11.4.A. Patient Rooms

11.4.A1. Patient room areas shall be 120 square feet (11.15 square meters) in single bedrooms and 200 square feet (18.58 square meters) in multiple-bed rooms.

11.4.A2. A nurses call system shall be provided in accordance with standards contained in Section 7.32.H. Provisions shall be made for easy removal or for covering call button outlets.

11.4.A3. Each patient bedroom shall have storage for extra blankets, pillows, and linen.

11.4.A4. Door to patient room shall be a minimum of 3 feet 8 inches wide (1.12 meters).

11.4.B. Service Areas

11.4.B1. Patients shall have access to at least one bathtub in each nursing unit.

11.4.B2. The standards of Section 11.2.B16 shall apply for social spaces except that the combined area for social activities shall be 30 square feet (2.79 square meters) per patient.

11.4.B3. Storage space for wheelchairs shall be provided in the nursing unit.

11.5 Forensic Psychiatric Unit

The standards of Section 11.2 shall be applied to forensic units. Forensic units shall have security vestibules or sally ports at the unit entrance. Specialized program requirements may indicate the need for additional treatment areas, police and courtroom space, and security considerations. Children, juveniles, and adolescents shall be separated from the adult areas.

11.6 Radiology Suite

Radiology services are not required to be provided within a psychiatric hospital. If they are provided within the hospital, the radiology suite shall comply with Section 7.10.

11.7 Nuclear Medicine

Nuclear medicine services are not required to be provided within a psychiatric hospital. If they are provided within the hospital, the nuclear medicine area shall comply with Section 7.11.

11.8 Laboratory Suite

Required laboratory tests may be performed on-site or provided through a contractual arrangement with a laboratory service.

Provisions shall be made for the following procedures to be performed on-site: urinalysis, blood glucose, and electrolytes. Provisions shall also be made for specimen collection and processing.

Minimum facilities on-site shall include a defined area with a laboratory lab counter, sink with water, refrigerated storage, storage for equipment and supplies, clerical area, and record storage.

11.9 Rehabilitation Therapy Department

11.9.A. General
Rehabilitation therapy in a psychiatric hospital is primarily for the diagnosis and treatment of mental functions but may also seek to address physical functions in varying degrees. It may contain one or several categories of services. If a formal rehabilitative therapy service is included in a project, the facilities and equipment shall be as necessary for the effective function of the program. Where two or more rehabilitative services are included, items may be shared, as appropriate.

11.9.B. Common Elements
Each rehabilitative therapy department shall include the following, which may be shared or provided as separate units for each service.

11.9.B1. Office and clerical space with provision for filing and retrieval of patient records.

11.9.B2. Where reception and control station(s) are required by the program, provision shall be made for visual control of waiting and activity areas. (This may be combined with office and clerical space.)

11.9.B3. Patient waiting area(s) out of traffic, with provision for wheelchairs. Patient waiting time for rehabilitation therapy should be minimized in a psychiatric hospital. The waiting area may be omitted if not required by the program.

11.9.B4. Patient toilets with handwashing facilities accessible to wheelchair patients.

11.9.B5. A conveniently accessible housekeeping room and service sink for housekeeping use.

11.9.B6. A secured area or cabinet within the vicinity of each work area for securing staff personal effects.

11.9.B7. Convenient access to toilets and lockers.

11.9.B8. Access to a demonstration-conference room.

11.9.C. Physical Therapy
The physical health of a person can have a direct effect on his or her mental health. Therefore, physical therapy may be desirable in a psychiatric hospital, especially for long-term care patients and elderly patients.

If physical therapy is part of the service, the following, at least, shall be included.

11.9.C1. Individual treatment area(s) with privacy screens or curtains. Each such space shall have not less than 60 square feet (5.58 square meters) of clear floor area.

11.9.C2. Handwashing facilities for staff either within or at each treatment space. (One handwashing facility may serve several treatment stations.)

11.9.C3. Exercise area and facilities.

11.9.C4. Clean linen and towel storage.

11.9.C5. Storage for equipment and supplies.

11.9.C6. Separate storage for soiled linen, towels, and supplies.

11.9.C7. Dressing areas, showers, and lockers for outpatients to be treated.

11.9.C8. Provisions shall be made for thermotherapy, diathermy, ultrasonics, and hydrotherapy when required by the functional program.

11.9.D. Occupational Therapy
Occupational therapy may include such activities as woodworking, leather tooling, art, needlework, painting, sewing, metalwork, and ceramics. The following, at least, shall be included:

11.9.D1. Work areas and counters suitable for wheelchair access.

11.9.D2. Handwashing facilities.

11.9.D3. Storage for supplies and equipment.

11.9.D4. Secured storage for potentially harmful supplies and equipment.

*11.9.D5. A separate room or alcove for a kiln.

11.9.D6. Remote electrical switching for potentially harmful equipment.

11.9.D7. Work areas should be sized for one therapy group at a time.

*11.9.D8. Display areas.

11.9.E. Vocational Therapy
Vocational therapy assists patients in the development and maintenance of productive work and interaction skills through the use of work tasks. These activities may occur in an industrial therapy workshop in another department or outdoors. If this service is provided, the following, at least, shall be included:

11.9.E1. Work areas suitable for wheelchair access.

11.9.E2. Handwashing facilities if required by the program.

11.9.E3. Storage for supplies and equipment.

11.9.E4. Secured storage for potentially harmful supplies and equipment.

11.9.E5. Remote electrical switching for potentially harmful equipment.

11.9.E6. Group work areas should be sized for one therapy group at a time.

11.9.F. Recreation Therapy
Recreation therapy assists patients in the development and maintenance of community living skills through the use of leisure-time activity tasks. These activities may occur in a recreation therapy department, in specialized facilities (e.g., gymnasium), multipurpose space in other areas (e.g., the nursing unit), or outdoors. The following, at least, shall be included:

11.9.F1. Activity areas suitable for wheelchair access.

11.9.F2. Handwashing facilities if required by the program.

11.9.F3. Storage for supplies and equipment.

11.9.F4. Secured storage for potentially harmful supplies and equipment.

11.9.F5. Remote electrical switching for potentially harmful equipment.

11.9.G. Education Therapy
Education therapy may be a program requirement, especially for children and adolescents. If the service is provided, the following, at least, shall be included.

11.9.G1. Classroom with student desks with 30 square feet (2.79 square meters) per desk with at least 150 square feet (13.94 square meters) per classroom.

11.9.G2. Desk and lockable storage for the teacher.

11.9.G3. Storage for supplies, equipment, and books.

11.10 Pharmacy

11.10.A. General
As described in the functional program, the size and type of services to be provided in the pharmacy will depend on the type of patients and illnesses treated, the type of drug distribution system used, the number of patients to be served, and the extent of shared or purchased services. This shall be described in the functional program. The pharmacy room or suite shall be located for convenient access, staff control, and security. Facilities and equipment shall be as necessary to accommodate the functions of the program and shall include provisions for procurement, storage, distribution, and recording of drugs and other pharmacy products. (Satellite facilities, if provided, shall include those items required by the program.)

11.11 Dietary Facilities

(See Section 7.18.)

11.12 Administration and Public Areas

(See Section 7.19.)

11.13 Medical Records

(See Section 7.20.)

11.14 Central Services

If only primary medical care is provided, central services may not be required or may be provided by countertop sterilizing/cleaning equipment. If decontamination and sterilization are required on-site, a full central services shall be provided (see Section 7.21).

11.15 General Storage

General storage room(s) with a total area of not less than 4 square feet (0.37 square meters) per inpatient bed shall be provided. Storage may be in separate, concentrated areas within the institution or in one or more individual buildings on-site. A portion of this storage may be provided off-site.

11.16 Linen Services

(See Section 7.23.)

11.17 Facilities for Cleaning and Sanitizing Carts

(See Section 7.24.)

11.18 Employee Facilities

(See Section 7.25.)

11.19 Housekeeping Room

(See Section 7.26.)

11.20 Engineering Service and Equipment Area

(See Section 7.27.)

11.21 Waste Processing Services

(See Section 7.30.C.)

11.22 General Standards for Details and Finishes

The standards of Section 11.22 shall comply with Section 7.28 with the following exceptions.

11.22.A.
The minimum door width for patient use access in new work shall be at least 3 feet (.91 meters).

11.22.B.
When grab bars are provided, the space between the bar and the wall should be filled to prevent a cord being tied around it for hanging. Bars, including those which are part of such fixtures as soap dishes, shall be sufficiently anchored to sustain a concentrated load of 250 pounds (113.4 kilograms).

11.23 Design and Construction, Including Fire-Resistant Standards

(See Section 7.29.)

11.24 Reserved

11.25 Reserved

11.26 Reserved

11.27 Reserved

11.28 Reserved

11.29 Reserved

11.30 Special Systems

11.30.A. General

11.30.A1. Prior to acceptance of the facility, all special systems shall be tested and operated to demonstrate to the owner or his designated representative that the installation and performance of these systems conform to design intent. Test results shall be documented for maintenance files.

11.30.A2. Upon completion of the special systems equipment installation contract, the owner shall be furnished with a complete set of manufacturers' operating, maintenance, and preventive maintenance instructions, a parts lists, and complete procurement information including equipment numbers and descriptions. Operating staff persons shall also be provided with instructions for proper operation of systems and equipment. Required information shall include all safety or code ratings as needed.

11.30.A3. Insulation shall be provided surrounding special system equipment to conserve energy, protect personnel, and reduce noise.

11.30.B. Elevators

11.30.B1. All buildings with patient facilities (such as bedrooms, dining rooms, or recreation areas) or services (such as diagnostic or therapeutic) located on other than the main entrance floor shall have electric or hydraulic elevators. Installation and testing of elevators shall comply with ANSI/ASME A17.1 for new construction and ANSI/ASME A17.3 for existing facilities. (See ASCE 7-93 for seismic design and control systems requirements for elevators.)

a. Elevators shall be equipped with a two-way automatic level-maintaining device with an accuracy of $\pm\frac{1}{4}$ inch ($\pm.64$ centimeters).

Psychiatric Hospital

b. Each elevator, except those for material handling, shall be equipped with an independent keyed switch for staff use for bypassing all landing button calls and responding to car button calls only.

c. Elevator call buttons shall be key controlled if required by the functional program, and controls shall not be activated by heat or smoke. Light beams, if used for operating door reopening devices without touch, shall be used in combination with door-edge safety devices and shall be interconnected with a system of smoke detectors. This is so that the light control feature will be overridden or disengaged should it encounter smoke at any landing.

11.30.B2. Field inspections and tests shall be made and the owner shall be furnished with written certification stating that the installation meets the requirements set forth in this section as well as all applicable safety regulations and codes.

11.30.C. Waste Processing Services

11.30.C1. Storage and disposal. Facilities shall be provided for sanitary storage and treatment or disposal of waste using techniques acceptable to the appropriate health and environmental authorities. The functional program shall stipulate the categories and volumes of waste for disposal and shall stipulate the methods of disposal for each.

11.30.C2. Medical waste. Medical waste shall be disposed of either by incineration or other approved technologies. Incinerators or other major disposal equipment may be shared by two or more institutions.

a. Incinerators or other major disposal equipment may also be used to dispose of other medical waste when local regulations permit. Equipment shall be designed for the actual quantity and type of waste to be destroyed and should meet all applicable regulations.

b. Incinerators with 50-pounds-per-hour or greater capacities shall be in a separate room or outdoors; those with lesser capacities may be located in a separate area within the facility boiler room. Rooms and areas containing incinerators shall have adequate space and facilities for incinerator charging and cleaning, as well as necessary clearances for work and maintenance. Provisions shall be made for operation, temporary storage, and disposal of materials so that odors and fumes do not drift back into occupied areas. Existing approved incinerator installations, which are not in separate rooms or outdoors, may remain unchanged provided they meet the above criteria.

c. The design and construction of incinerators and trash chutes shall comply with NFPA 82.

*d. Heat recovery.

*e. Environmental guidelines.

11.31 Mechanical Standards

11.31.A. General

11.31.A1. The mechanical system should be designed for overall efficiency and appropriate life-cycle cost. Details for cost-effective implementation of design features are interrelated and too numerous (as well as too basic) to list individually. Recognized engineering procedures shall be followed for the most economical and effective results. A well-designed system can generally achieve energy efficiency at minimal additional cost and simultaneously provide improved patient comfort. Different geographic areas may have climatic and use conditions that favor one system over another in terms of overall cost and efficiency. In no case shall patient care or safety be sacrificed for conservation.

Mechanical, electrical, and HVAC equipment may be located either internally, externally, or in separate buildings.

11.31.A2. Remodeling and work in existing facilities may present special problems. As practicality and funding permit, existing insulation, weather stripping, etc., should be brought up to standard for maximum economy and efficiency. Consideration shall be given to additional work that may be needed to achieve this.

11.31.A3. Facility design consideration shall include site, building mass, orientation, configuration, fenestration, and other features relative to passive and active energy systems.

11.31.A4. Insofar as practical, the facility should include provisions for recovery of waste cooling and heating energy (ventilation, exhaust, water and steam discharge, cooling towers, incinerators, etc.).

11.31.A5. Facility design considerations shall include recognized energy-saving mechanisms such as variable-air-volume systems, load shedding, programmed controls for unoccupied periods (nights and weekends, etc.) and use of natural ventilation, site and climatic conditions permitting. Systems with excessive installation and/or maintenance costs that negate long-range energy savings should be avoided.

11.31.A6. Air-handling systems shall be designed with an economizer cycle where appropriate to use outside air. Use of mechanically circulated outside air does not reduce the need for filtration.

11.31.A.7. Mechanical equipment, ductwork, and piping shall be mounted on vibration isolators as required to prevent unacceptable structure-borne vibration.

11.31.A8. Supply and return mains and risers for cooling, heating, and steam systems shall be equipped with valves to isolate the various sections of each system. Each piece of equipment shall have valves at the supply and return ends.

11.31.B. Thermal and Acoustical Insulation

11.31.B1. Insulation within the building shall be provided to conserve energy, protect personnel, prevent vapor condensation, and reduce noise.

11.31.B2. Insulation on cold surfaces shall include an exterior vapor barrier. (Material that will not absorb or transmit moisture will not require a separate vapor barrier.)

11.31.B3. Insulation, including finishes and adhesives on the exterior surfaces of ducts, piping, and equipment, shall have a flame-spread rating of 25 or less and a smoke-developed rating of 50 or less as determined by an independent testing laboratory in accordance with NFPA 255.

11.31.B4. If duct lining is used, it shall be coated and sealed, and shall meet ASTM C1071. These linings (including coatings, adhesives, and exterior surface insulation on pipes and ducts in spaces used as air supply plenums) shall have a flame-spread rating of 25 or less and a smoke-developed rating of 50 or less, as determined by an independent testing laboratory in accordance with NFPA 255. If existing lined ductwork is reworked in a renovation project, the liner seams and punctures shall be resealed.

11.31.B5. Existing accessible insulation within areas of facilities to be modernized shall be inspected, repaired, and/or replaced, as appropriate.

11.31.B6. Duct lining shall not be installed within 15 feet (4.57 meters) downstream of humidifiers.

11.31.C. Steam and Hot Water Systems

11.31.C1. Boilers shall have the capacity, based upon the net ratings published by the Hydronics Institute or another acceptable national standard, to supply the normal heating, hot water, and steam requirements of all systems and equipment.

11.31.D. Air Conditioning, Heating, and Ventilation Systems

11.31.D1. All rooms and areas in the facility used for patient care shall have provisions for ventilation. The ventilation rates shown in Table 2 shall be used only as minimum standards; they do not preclude the use of higher, more appropriate rates. Fans serving exhaust systems shall be located at the discharge end and shall be readily serviceable. Air supply and exhaust in rooms for which no minimum total air change rate is noted may vary down to zero in response to room load. For rooms listed in Table 2, where VAV systems are used, minimum total air change shall be within limits noted. Temperature control shall also comply with these standards. The ventilation systems shall be designed and balanced according to the requirements shown in Table 2 and in the applicable notes.

11.31.D2. General exhaust systems may be combined to enhance the efficiency of recovery devices required for energy conservation. Local exhaust systems shall be used whenever possible in place of dilution ventilation to reduce exposure to hazardous gases, vapors, fumes, or mists.

11.31.D3. Fresh air intakes shall be located at least 25 feet (7.62 meters) from exhaust outlets of ventilating systems, combustion equipment stacks, medical-surgical vacuum systems, plumbing vents, or areas that may collect vehicular exhaust or other noxious fumes. (Prevailing winds and/or proximity to other structures may require greater clearances.) Plumbing and vacuum vents that terminate at a level above the top of the air intake may be located as close as 10 feet (3.05 meters). The bottom of outdoor air intakes serving central systems shall be as high as practical, but at least 6 feet (1.83 meters) above ground level, or, if installed above the roof, 3 feet (.91 meter) above roof level. Exhaust outlets from areas that may be contaminated shall be above roof level, arranged to minimize recirculation of exhaust air into the building, and directed away from personnel service areas.

11.31.D4. All central ventilation or air conditioning systems shall be equipped with filters with efficiencies equal to, or greater than, those specified in Table 11. Filter efficiencies, tested in accordance with ASHRAE 52-92, shall be average. Filter frames shall be durable and proportioned to provide an airtight fit with the enclosing ductwork. All joints between filter segments and enclosing ductwork shall have gaskets or seals to provide a positive seal against air leakage. A manometer shall be installed across each filter bed having a required efficiency of 75 percent or more.

*11.31.D5. If duct humidifiers are located upstream of the final filters, they shall be located at least 15 feet (4.57 meters) upstream of the final filters. Ductwork with duct-mounted humidifiers shall have a means of water removal. An adjustable high-limit humidistat shall be located downstream of the humidifier to reduce the potential for condensation inside the duct. All duct takeoffs shall be sufficiently downstream of the humidifier to ensure complete moisture absorption. Steam humidifiers shall be used. Reservoir-type water spray or evaporative pan humidifiers shall not be used.

11.31.D6. Air-handling duct systems shall be designed with accessibility for duct cleaning, and shall meet the requirements of NFPA 90A.

11.31.D7. Ducts that penetrate construction intended for X-ray or other ray protection shall not impair the effectiveness of the protection.

11.31.D8. Fire and smoke dampers shall be constructed, located, and installed in accordance with the requirements of NFPA 101, 90A, and the specific damper's Listing requirements. Fans, dampers, and detectors shall be interconnected so that damper activation will not damage ducts. Maintenance access shall be provided at all dampers. All damper locations should be shown on design drawings. Dampers should be activated by fire or smoke sensors, not by fan cutoff alone. Switching systems for restarting fans may be installed for fire department use in venting smoke after a fire has been controlled. However, provisions should be made to avoid possible damage to the system due to closed dampers. When smoke partitions are required, heating, ventilation, and air conditioning zones shall be coordinated with compartmentation insofar as practical to minimize the need to penetrate fire and smoke partitions.

11.31.D9. Exhaust hoods handling grease-laden vapors in food preparation centers shall comply with NFPA 96. All hoods over cooking ranges shall be equipped with grease filters, fire extinguishing systems, and heat-actuated fan controls. Cleanout openings shall be provided every 20 feet (6.10 meters), and at changes in direction in the horizontal exhaust duct systems serving these hoods. (Horizontal runs of ducts serving range hoods should be kept to a minimum.)

11.31.D10. Rooms with fuel-fired equipment shall be provided with sufficient outdoor air to maintain equipment combustion rates and to limit work station temperatures.

11.31.D11. Gravity exhaust may be used, where conditions permit, for nonpatient areas such as boiler rooms, central storage, etc.

11.31.D12. The energy-saving potential of variable air volume systems is recognized and these standards herein are intended to maximize appropriate use of that system. Any system utilized for occupied areas shall include provisions to avoid air stagnation in interior spaces where thermostat demands are met by temperatures of surrounding areas.

11.31.D13. Special consideration shall be given to the type of heating and cooling units, ventilation outlets, and appurtenances installed in patient-occupied areas. The following shall apply:

a. All air grilles and diffusers shall be of a type that prohibits the insertion of foreign objects. All exposed fasteners shall be tamper-resistant.

b. All convector or HVAC enclosures exposed in the room shall be constructed with rounded corners and shall have enclosures fastened with tamper-resistant screws.

c. HVAC equipment shall be of a type that minimizes the need for maintenance within the room.

*11.31.D14. Rooms or booths used for sputum induction, aerosolized pentamidine treatments, and other high-risk cough-inducing procedures shall be provided with local exhaust ventilation.

11.31.D15. Non-central air-handling systems, i.e., individual room units used for heating and cooling purposes (fan-coil units, heat pump units, etc.) shall be equipped with permanent (cleanable) or replaceable filters. The filters shall have a minimum efficiency of 68 percent weight arrestance. These units may be used as recirculating units only. All outdoor requirements shall be met by a separate central air-handling system with the proper filtration, as noted in Table 11.

11.31.E. Plumbing and Other Piping Systems

Unless otherwise specified herein, all plumbing systems shall be designed and installed in accordance with the National Standard Plumbing Code, chapter 14, Medical Care Facility Plumbing Equipment.

11.31.E1. The following standards shall apply to plumbing fixtures:

a. The material used for plumbing fixtures shall be nonabsorptive and acid-resistant.

b. Waterspouts used in lavatories and sinks shall have clearances adequate to avoid contaminating utensils and the contents of carafes, etc.

c. General handwashing facilities used by medical and nursing staff and all lavatories used by patients and food handlers shall be trimmed with valves that can be operated without hands. (Single lever or wrist blade devices may be used.) Blade handles used for this purpose shall not exceed 4½ inches (11.43 cm) in length. Handles on clinical sinks shall be at least 6 inches (15.24 cm) long. Freestanding scrub sinks and lavatories used for scrubbing in procedure rooms shall be trimmed with foot, knee, or ultrasonic controls (no single-lever wrist blades).

d. Clinical sinks shall have an integral trap wherein the upper portion of the water trap provides a visible seal.

e. Showers and tubs shall have nonslip walking surfaces.

11.31.E2. The following standards shall apply to potable water supply systems:

a. Systems shall be designed to supply water at sufficient pressure to operate all fixtures and equipment during maximum demand. Supply capacity for hot- and cold-water piping shall be determined on the basis of fixture units, using recognized engineering standards. When the ratio of plumbing fixtures to occupants is proportionally more than required by the building occupancy and is in excess of 1,000 plumbing fixture units, a diversity factor is permitted.

b. Each water service main, branch main, riser, and branch to a group of fixtures shall have valves. Stop valves shall be provided for each fixture. Appropriate panels for access shall be provided at all valves where required.

c. Vacuum breakers shall be installed on hose bibs and supply nozzles used for connection of hoses or tubing in laboratories, housekeeping sinks, bedpan-flushing attachments, and autopsy tables, etc.

d. Bedpan-flushing devices (may be cold water) shall be provided in each inpatient toilet room; however, installation is optional in psychiatric and alcohol-abuse units where patients are ambulatory.

e. Potable water storage vessels (hot and cold) not intended for constant use shall not be installed.

11.31.E3. The following standards shall apply to hot water systems:

a. The water-heating system shall have sufficient supply capacity at the temperatures and amounts indicated in Table 4. Water temperature is measured at the point of use or inlet to the equipment.

b. Hot-water distribution systems serving patient care areas shall be under constant recirculation to provide continuous hot water at each hot water outlet. The temperature of hot water for showers and bathing shall be appropriate for comfortable use but shall not exceed 110°F (43°C) (see Table 4).

11.31.E4. The following standards shall apply to drainage systems:

a. Drain lines from sinks used for acid waste disposal shall be made of acid-resistant material.

b. Drain lines serving some types of automatic blood-cell counters must be of carefully selected material that will eliminate potential for undesirable chemical reactions (and/or explosions) between sodium azide wastes and copper, lead, brass, and solder, etc.

c. Insofar as possible, drainage piping shall not be installed within the ceiling or exposed in food preparation centers, food serving facilities, food storage areas, central services, electronic data processing areas, electric closets, and other sensitive areas. Where exposed, overhead drain piping in these areas is unavoidable, special provisions shall be made to protect the space below from leakage, condensation, or dust particles.

d. Floor drains shall not be installed in operating rooms.

e. Drain systems for autopsy tables shall be designed to positively avoid splatter or overflow onto floors or back siphonage and for easy cleaning and trap flushing.

f. Building sewers shall discharge into community sewerage. Where such a system is not available, the facility shall treat its sewage in accordance with local and state regulations.

g. Kitchen grease traps shall be located and arranged to permit easy access without the need to enter food preparation or storage areas. Grease traps shall be of the capacity required and shall be accessible from outside of building without the need to interrupt any services.

h. In dietary areas, floor drains and/or floor sinks shall be of a type that can be easily cleaned by removing the cover. Provide floor drains or floor sinks at all "wet" equipment (as ice machines) and as required for wet cleaning of floors. Provide removable stainless steel mesh in addition to grilled drain covers to prevent entry of large particles of waste that might cause stoppages. Location of floor drains and floor sinks shall be coordinated to avoid conditions in which locations of equipment make removal of covers for cleaning difficult.

11.31.E5. The installation, testing, and certification of nonflammable medical gas and air systems shall comply with the requirements of NFPA 99. (See Table 5 for rooms requiring station outlets.)

11.31.E6. Clinical vacuum system installations shall be in accordance with NFPA 99. (See Table 5 for rooms which require station outlets.)

11.31.E7. All piping, except control-line tubing, shall be identified. All valves shall be tagged, and a valve schedule shall be provided to the facility owner for permanent record and reference.

11.31.E8. Provide condensate drains for cooling coils of a type that may be cleaned as needed without disassembly. (Unless specifically required by local authorities, traps are not required for condensate drains.) Provide an air gap where condensate drains empty into floor drains. Provide heater elements for condensate lines in freezers or other areas where freezing may be a problem.

11.31.E9. No plumbing lines may be exposed overhead or on walls where possible accumulation of dust or soil may create a cleaning problem or where leaks would create a potential for food contamination.

11.32. Electrical Standards

11.32.A. General

11.32.A1. All electrical material and equipment, including conductors, controls, and signaling devices, shall be installed in compliance with applicable sections of NFPA 70 and NFPA 99 and shall be listed as complying with available standards of listing agencies or other similar established standards when such standards are required.

11.32.A2. The electrical installations, including alarm, nurse call, staff emergency signed system, and communication systems, shall be tested to demonstrate that equipment installation and operation is appropriate and functional. A written record of performance tests on special electrical systems and equipment shall show compliance with applicable codes and standards.

11.32.A3. Data processing and/or automated laboratory or diagnostic equipment, if provided, may require safeguards from power line disturbances.

11.32.B. Services and Switchboards

Main switchboards shall be located in an area separate from plumbing and mechanical equipment and shall be accessible to authorized persons only. Switchboards shall be convenient for use, readily accessible for maintenance, away from traffic lanes, and located in dry, ventilated spaces free of corrosive or explosive fumes, gases, or any flammable material. Overload protective devices shall operate properly in ambient room temperatures.

11.32.C. Panelboards

Panelboards serving normal lighting and appliance circuits shall be located on the same floor as the circuits they serve. Panelboards serving critical branch emergency circuits shall be located on each floor that has major users. Panelboards serving Life Safety emergency circuits may also serve floors above and/or below.

11.32.D. Lighting

11.32.D1. Lighting shall be engineered to the specific application.

11.32.D2. The Illuminating Engineering Society of North America (IES) has developed recommended lighting levels for health care facilities. The reader should refer to the *IES Handbook* (1993).

11.32.D3. Approaches to buildings and parking lots and all occupied spaces shall have fixtures for lighting that can be illuminated as necessary.

11.32.D4. Patient rooms shall have general lighting and night lighting. At least one night light fixture in each patient room shall be controlled at the room entrance.

11.32.D5. Nursing unit corridors shall have general illumination with provisions for reducing light levels at night.

11.32.D6. Consideration should be given to the special needs of the elderly. Excessive contrast in lighting levels that makes effective sight adaptation difficult should be minimized.

11.32.E. Receptacles (Convenience Outlets)

11.32.E1. Each patient room shall have duplex-grounded receptacles. There shall be one at each side of the head of each bed and one on every other wall. Receptacles may be omitted from exterior walls when construction or room configuration makes installation impractical. These outlets shall be tamper-resistant or equipped with ground-fault circuit interrupters (GFCIs).

11.32.E2. Duplex-grounded receptacles for general use shall be installed approximately 50 feet (15.24 meters) apart in all corridors and within 25 feet (7.62 meters) of corridor ends. These outlets shall be tamper-resistant or equipped with GFCIs.

11.32.E3. Electrical receptacle coverplates or electrical receptacles supplied from the emergency system shall be distinctively colored or marked for identification. If color is used for identification purposes, the same color should be used throughout the facility.

11.32.F. Equipment

11.32.F1. Ground-fault circuit interrupters shall comply with NFPA 70. When GFCIs are used in critical areas, provisions shall be made to ensure that other essential equipment is not affected by activation of one interrupter.

11.32.F2. Special equipment is identified in the following sections: Nursing Units, Resident Support Areas, Rehabilitation Therapy, Laboratory, Pharmacy, and Imaging, if applicable. These sections shall be consulted to ensure compatibility between programmatically defined equipment needs and appropriate power and other electrical connection needs.

11.32.G. Nurse Calling System

11.32.G1. A nurses calling system is not required in psychiatric nursing units, but if it is included provisions shall be made for easy removal or for covering call buttons. All hardware shall have tamper-resistant fasteners. Calls shall activate a visible signal in the corridor at the patient's door and at an annunciator panel at the nurse station or other appropriate location. In multicorridor nursing units, additional visible signals shall be installed at corridor intersections.

11.32.G2. The staff emergency call, if provided, shall be designed so that a signal activated by staff at a patient's calling station will initiate a visible and audible signal distinct from the regular nurse calling system. The signal shall activate an annunciator panel at the nurses station or other appropriate location, a distinct visible signal in the corridor at the door to the room from which the signal was initiated, and at other areas defined by the functional program.

11.32.G3. Alternate technologies can be considered for emergency or nurse call systems. If radio frequency systems are utilized, consideration should be given to electromagnetic compatibility between internal and external sources.

11.32.H. Emergency Electrical Service

11.32.H1. As a minimum, nursing facilities or sections thereof shall have emergency electrical systems as required in NFPA 101, NFPA 110, and NFPA 99.

11.32.H2. When the psychiatric facility is a distinct part of an acute-care hospital, it may use the emergency generator system for required emergency lighting and power, if such sharing does not reduce hospital services. Life support systems and their respective areas shall be subject to applicable standards of Section 7.32.

11.32.H3. An emergency electrical source shall provide lighting and/or power during an interruption of the normal electric supply.

11.32.I. Fire Alarm System
Fire alarm and detection systems shall be provided in compliance with NFPA 101 and NFPA 72.

11.32.J. Telecommunications and Information Systems

11.32.J1. Locations for terminating telecommunications and information system devices shall be provided.

11.32.J2. An area shall be provided for central equipment locations. Special air conditioning and voltage regulation shall be provided when recommended by the manufacturer.

Table 11

Filter Efficiencies for Central Ventilation and Air Conditioning Systems in Psychiatric Hospitals

Area Designation	Mininum number of filter beds	Filter efficiencies (%)	
		Filter bed no. 1	Filter bed no. 2
All areas for inpatient care, treatment, and diagnosis, and those areas providing direct service	2	30	90
Administrative, bulk storage, soiled holding, laundries, food preparation areas	1	30	—

Note: Filtration efficiency ratings are based on dust spot efficiency per ASHRAE 52–92.

12. MOBILE, TRANSPORTABLE, AND RELOCATABLE UNITS

12.1 General

12.1.A. Application
This section applies to mobile, transportable, and relocatable structures. The size of these units limits occupancy, thereby minimizing hazards and allowing for less stringent standards. Needed community services can therefore be provided at an affordable cost. These facilities shall be defined as space and equipment service for four or fewer workers at any one time. Meeting all provisions of Section 9.2 for general outpatient facilities is desirable, but limited size and resources may preclude satisfying any but the basic minimums described. Specifically described are:

12.1.A1. Mobile units.

12.1.A2. Transportable units.

12.1.A3. Relocatable units.

12.1.B. Definitions

12.1.B1. Mobile unit.
Any premanufactured structure, trailer, or self-propelled unit equipped with a chassis on wheels and intended to provide shared medical services to the community on a temporary basis. These units are typically 8 feet wide by 48 feet long (2.44 meters by 14.63 meters) (or less), some equipped with expanding walls, and designed to be moved on a daily basis.

12.1.B2. Transportable unit.
Any premanufactured structure or trailer, equipped with a chassis on wheels, intended to provide shared medical services to the community on an extended temporary basis. The units are typically 12 feet wide by 60 feet long (3.66 meters by 18.29 meters) (or less) and are designed to move periodically, depending on need.

12.1.B3. Relocatable unit.
Any structure, not on wheels, built to be relocated at any time and provide medical services. These structures vary in size.

12.1.C. Classification
The classifications of these facilities shall be Business Occupancy as listed in the building codes and NFPA 101 Life Safety Code.

Units shall comply with NFPA 101 where patients incapable of self-preservation or those receiving inhalation anesthesia are treated.

12.1.D. Common Elements for Mobile, Transportable, and Relocatable Units

12.1.D1. Site conditions.

a. Access for the unit to arrive shall be taken into consideration for space planning. Turning radius of the vehicles, slopes of the approach (6 percent maximum), and existing conditions shall be addressed.

b. Gauss fields of various strengths of magnetic resonance imaging (MRI) units shall be considered for the environmental effect on the field homogeneity and vice versa. Radio frequency interference shall be considered when planning the site.

c. Sites shall be provided with properly sized power, including emergency power, water, waste, telephone, and fire alarm connections, as required by local and state building codes.

d. Sites shall have level concrete pads or piers and be designed for the structural loads of the facility. Construction of pads shall meet local, state, and seismic codes. Concrete-filled steel pipe bollards are recommended for protection of the facility and the unit.

e. Sites utilizing MRI systems shall consider providing adequate access for cryogen-servicing of the magnet. Cryogen dewars are of substantial weight and size. Storage of dewars also shall be included in space planning.

f. It is recommended that each site provide a covered walkway or enclosure to ensure patient safety from the outside elements.

g. Consideration shall be given to location of the unit so that diesel exhaust of the tractor and/or unit generator is kept away from the fresh air intake of the facility.

h. It is recommended that each facility provide a means of preventing unit movement, either by blocking the wheels or by providing pad anchors.

i. Sites shall provide hazard-free drop-off zones and adequate parking for patients.

j. The facility shall provide waiting space for patient privacy and patient/staff toilets as close to the unit docking area as possible.

k. Each site shall provide access to the unit for wheelchair/stretcher patients.

l. Mobile units shall be provided with handwashing facilities unless each site can provide handwashing facilities within a 25-foot (7.62 meter) proximity to the unit. Transportable and relocatable units shall be provided with handwashing facilities.

m. It is recommended that each site requiring water and waste services to the unit provide a means of freeze protection in geographical areas where freezing temperatures occur.

12.1.D2. Site considerations—relocatable units. Seismic force resistance for relocatable units shall comply with Section 1.4 and shall be given an importance factor of one when applied to the seismic design formulas. These units shall meet the structural requirements of the local and state building codes.

12.1.E. General Standards for Details and Finishes for Unit Construction

12.1.E1. Existing facilities.
Existing facilities shall comply with applicable requirements of the existing Business Occupancies, Chapter 27, of NFPA 101; and where there are patients incapable of self-preservation receiving inhalation anesthesia, existing Ambulatory Health Care Centers, Chapter 13-6, shall apply.

12.1.E2. Details and finishes.
Requirements below apply to all units unless noted otherwise:

a. Horizontal sliding doors and power-operated doors shall comply with NFPA 101.

b. Units shall be permitted a single means of egress as permitted by NFPA 101.

c. All glazing in doors shall be safety or wire glass.

d. Stairs for mobile and transportable units shall be in accordance with the following table:

New units

Minimum width clear of all obstructions, except projections not exceeding 3½ inches at or below handrail height on each side	34 inches (86.36 centimeters)
Minimum headroom	6 ft. 8 inches (2.03 meters)
Maximum height of risers	9 inches (22.86 centimeters)
Minimum height of risers	4 inches (10.16 centimeters)
Minimum tread depth	9 inches (22.86 centimeters)
Doors opening immediately onto stairs without a landing	NO

Existing units

Minimum width clear of all obstructions, except projections not exceeding 3½ inches at or below handrail height on each side	27 inches (.69 meters)
Minimum headroom	6 ft. 8 inches (2.03 meters)
Maximum height of risers	9 inches (22.86 centimeters)
Minimum height of risers	4 inches (10.16 centimeters)
Minimum tread depth	7 inches (17.78 centimeters)
Doors opening immediately onto stairs without a landing	YES

There shall be no variation exceeding 3/16 inch in depth of adjacent treads or in the height of adjacent risers, and the tolerance between the largest and smallest tread shall not exceed 3/8 inch in any flight.

Exception: When the bottom riser adjoins a public way, walk, or driveway having an established grade and serving as a landing, a variation in height of not more than 3 inches (0.08 meter) in every 3 feet (0.91 meter) and fraction of thereafter is permitted. Adjustable legs at the bottom of the stair assembly shall be permitted to allow for grade differences.

Stairs and landings for relocatable units shall comply with NFPA 101.

e. Handrails shall be provided on at least one side. Handrails shall be installed and constructed in accordance with NFPA 101, with the following exception: Provided the distance from grade to unit floor height is not greater than 4 feet 5 inches (1.35 meters), one intermediate handrail, having clear distance between rails of 19 inches (0.48 meter) maximum, shall be permitted. Exception: Existing units having a floor height of 63 inches (1.60 meters) maximum.

f. All units shall be equipped with an automatic sprinkler system or other automatic extinguishing equipment as defined in NFPA 101. In addition, manual fire extinguishers shall be provided in accordance with NFPA 101. Exception: Existing units equipped with portable fire extinguishers.

g. Fire detection, alarm, and communications capabilities shall be installed and connected to the facility's central alarm system on all new units in accordance with NFPA 101.

h. Radiation protection for X-ray and gamma ray installations shall be in accordance with NCRP reports numbers 49 and 91 in addition to all applicable local and state requirements.

i. Interior finish materials shall be class A as defined in NFPA 101.

j. Textile materials having a napped, tufted, looped, woven, nonwoven, or similar surface shall be permitted on walls and ceilings provided such materials have a class "A" rating and rooms or areas are protected by an automatic extinguishment or sprinkler system.

k. Fire retardant coatings shall be permitted in accordance with NFPA 101.

l. Curtains and draperies shall be noncombustible or flame retardant and shall pass both the large and small scale tests required by NFPA 101.

12.1.F. Environmental Standards
All mobile, transportable, and relocatable units shall be sited in full compliance with such federal, state, and local environmental laws and regulations as may apply, for example, those listed in Section 3.3.

12.2 Reserved

12.3 Reserved

12.4 Reserved

12.5 Reserved

12.6 Reserved

12.7 Reserved

12.8 Reserved

12.9 Reserved

12.10 Reserved

12.11 Reserved

12.12 Reserved

12.13 Reserved

12.14 Reserved

12.15 Reserved

12.16 Reserved

12.17 Reserved

12.18 Reserved

12.19 Reserved

12.20 Reserved

12.21 Reserved

12.22 Reserved

12.23 Reserved

12.24 Reserved

12.25 Reserved

12.26 Reserved

12.27 Reserved

12.28 Reserved

12.29 Reserved

12.30 Reserved

12.31. Mechanical Standards

12.31.A.
Air conditioning, heating, ventilating, ductwork, and related equipment shall be installed in accordance with NFPA 90A, Standard for the Installation of Air Conditioning and Ventilation systems.

12.31.B.
All other requirements for heating and ventilation systems shall comply with Sections 9.31.A through 9.31.D.

12.31.C. Plumbing Standards

12.31.C1. Plumbing and other piping systems shall be installed in accordance with applicable model plumbing codes, unless specified herein.

12.31.C2. Mobile units, requiring sinks, shall not be required to be vented through the roof. Ventilation of waste lines shall be permitted to be vented through the sidewalls or other acceptable locations. Transportable and relocatable units shall be vented through the roof per model plumbing codes.

12.31.C3. All waste lines shall be designed and constructed to discharge into the facility sanitary sewage system.

12.31.C4. Backflow prevention shall be installed at the point of water connection on the unit.

12.31.C5. Medical gases and suction systems, if installed, shall be in accordance with NFPA 99.

12.32. Electrical Standards

12.32.A. General

12.32.A1. All electrical material and equipment, including conductors, controls, and signaling devices, shall be installed in compliance with applicable sections of NFPA 70 and NFPA 99 and shall be listed as complying with available standards of listing agencies or other similar established standards where such standards are required.

12.32.A2. The electrical installations, including alarm, nurse call, and communication systems, shall be tested to demonstrate that equipment installation and operation is appropriate and functional. A written record of performance tests on special electrical systems and equipment shall show compliance with applicable codes and standards.

12.32.A3. Data processing and/or automated laboratory or diagnostic equipment, if provided, may require safeguards from power line disturbances.

12.32.B. Services and Switchboards

Main switchboards shall be located in an area separate from plumbing and mechanical equipment and shall be accessible to authorized persons only. Switchboards shall be convenient for use, readily accessible for maintenance, away from traffic lanes, and located in dry, ventilated spaces free of corrosive or explosive fumes, gases, or any flammable material. Overload protective devices shall operate properly in ambient room temperatures.

12.32.C. Panelboards

Panelboards serving normal lighting and appliance circuits shall be located on the same level as the circuits they serve.

12.32.D. Lighting

12.32.D1. Lighting shall be engineered to the specific application.

12.32.D2. The Illuminating Engineering Society of North America (IES) has developed recommended lighting levels for health care facilities. The reader should refer to the *IES Handbook* (1993).

12.32.D3. Approaches to buildings and parking lots and all occupied spaces shall have fixtures for lighting that can be illuminated as necessary.

12.32.D4. Consideration should be given to the special needs of the elderly. Excessive contrast in lighting levels that makes effective sight adaptation difficult should be minimized.

12.32.D5. A portable or fixed examination light shall be provided for examination, treatment, and trauma rooms.

12.32.E. Receptacles (Convenience Outlets)

Duplex grounded-type receptacles (convenience outlets) shall be installed in all areas in sufficient quantities for tasks to be performed as needed. Each examination and work table shall have access to a minimum of two duplex receptacles.

12.32.F. Equipment

12.32.F1. At inhalation anesthetizing locations, all electrical equipment and devices, receptacles, and wiring shall comply with applicable sections of NFPA 99 and NFPA 70.

12.32.F2. Fixed and mobile X-ray equipment installations shall conform to articles 517 and 660 of NFPA 70.

12.32.G. Reserved

12.32.H. Emergency Electrical Service

Emergency lighting and power shall be provided for in accordance with NFPA 99, NFPA 101, and NFPA 110.

12.32.I. Fire Alarm System

The fire alarm system shall be as described in NFPA 101 and where applicable NFPA 72.

12.32.J. Telecommunications and Information Systems

12.32.J1. Locations for terminating telecommunications and information system devices shall be located on the unit that the devices serve and shall be accessible to authorized personnel only.

12.32.J2. Special air conditioning and voltage regulation shall be provided when recommended by the manufacturer.

*13. HOSPICE CARE

APPENDIX A

This appendix is not part of the requirements of these Guidelines, but is included for information purposes only.

The following notes, bearing the same number as the text of the Guidelines to which they apply, contain useful explanatory material and references.

A1.4

Owners of existing facilities should undertake an assessment of their facility with respect to its ability to withstand the effects of regional natural disasters. The assessment should consider performance of structural and critical nonstructural building systems and the likelihood of loss of externally supplied power, gas, water, and communications under such conditions. Facility master planning should consider mitigation measures required to address conditions that may be hazardous to patients and conditions that may compromise the ability of the facility to fulfill its planned post- emergency medical response. Particular attention should be paid to seismic considerations in areas where the effective peak acceleration coefficient, Aa, of ASCE 7-93 exceeds 0.15.

A1.4.A.

The ASCE 7-93 seismic provisions are based on the National Earthquake Hazards Reduction Program (NEHRP) provisions (1988 edition) developed by the Building Seismic Safety Council (BSSC) for the Federal Emergency Management Agency (FEMA).

A study by the National Institute of Standards and Technology (NIST) found that the following seismic standards were essentially equivalent to the NEHRP (1988) provisions:

- 1991 ICBO Uniform Building Code

- 1992 Supplement to the BOCA National Building Code

- 1992 Amendments to the SBCC Standard Building Code

Executive Order 12699, dated January 5, 1990, specified the use of the maps in the most recent edition of ANSI A58 for seismic safety of federal and federally assisted or regulated new building construction. The ASCF 7 standard was formerly the ANSI A58 standard. Public Law 101-614 charged FEMA to "prepare and disseminate widely....information on building codes and practices for buildings..." The NEHRP provisions were developed to provide this guidance.

A3.1.B. Availability of Transportation

Facilities should be located so that they are convenient to public transportation where it is available, unless acceptable alternate methods of transportation to public facilities and services are provided.

A4.1.B.

Design should consider the placement of cables from portable equipment so that circulation and safety are maintained.

A4.2.C1. Examples of movable equipment include operating tables, treatment and examination tables, laboratory centrifuges, food service trucks and other wheeled carts, and patient room furnishings.

A4.3 Major Technical Equipment

Examples of major technical equipment are X-ray and other imaging equipment, radiation therapy equipment, lithotripters, audiometry testing chambers, laundry equipment, computers, and similar items.

A.5.1.

Partitions and enclosures around renovation areas should be solid in nature, securely attached, and sealed at the floor and structure above. Where life safety does not warrant special constructions, measures should be taken to control the transmission of dust and other airborne substances. One method for achieving this is by means of a separate ventilation/exhaust system for the construction area, thereby maintaining negative air pressure in the construction area. This would require further documentation of locations of fresh air intakes and filters (where necessary), as well as the disconnection of existing air ducts, as required.

A.5.2.

Particular attention should be paid to areas requiring special ventilation, including surgical services, protective environment rooms, airborne infection isolation rooms, laboratories, autopsy rooms, and local exhaust systems for hazardous agents. These areas should be recognized as needing mechanical systems that comply with infection control and/or laboratory safety requirements.

A7.1.E.
Facility design for swing beds often requires additional corridor doors and provisions for switching nurse call operations from one nurse station to another depending on use.

A7.2.A2. These areas are recognized as minimums and do not prohibit the use of larger rooms when required for needs and functions. The degree of acuteness of care being provided should be the determining factor.

A7.2.A3. Windows are important for the psychological well-being of many patients, as well as for meeting fire safety code requirements. They are also essential for continued use of the area in the event of mechanical ventilation system failure.

A7.2.A4. A handwashing facility may be provided in the patient room in addition to that in the toilet room. This facility should be located near the patient room entrance door.

A7.2.D.
Immunosuppressed Host Airborne Infection Isolation (Protective Environment/Airborne Infection Isolation). An anteroom is required for the special case in which an immunosuppressed patient requires airborne infection isolation. Immunosuppression is defined in 7.2.D. There is no prescribed method for anteroom ventilation—the room can be ventilated with either of the following airflow patterns: (a) airflows from the anteroom, to the patient room and the corridor, or (b) airflows from the patient room and the corridor, into the anteroom. The advantage of pattern (a) is the provision for a clean anteroom in which health care workers need not mask before entering the anteroom.

A7.3.A2. Transportation of patients to and from the critical care unit should ideally be separated from public corridors and visitor waiting areas. In new construction, where elevator transport is required for critically ill patients, the size of the cab and mechanisms and controls should meet the specialized needs.

A7.3.A3. In critical care units, the size of the patient care space should depend on the intended functional use. The patient space in critical care units, especially those caring for surgical patients following major trauma or cardiovascular, transplant, or orthopedic procedures, or medical patients simultaneously requiring ventilation, dialysis, and/or other large equipment (e.g., intra-aortic balloon pump) may be overwhelmed if designed to the absolute minimum clear floor area.

A staff emergency assistance system should be provided on the most accessible side of the bed. The system should annunciate at the nurse station with backup from another staffed area from which assistance can be summoned.

Provision should be made for rapid and easily accessible information exchange and communication within the unit and the hospital.

The unit should provide the ability to continuously monitor the physiological parameters appropriate for the types of patients the unit is expected to care for.

A7.3.A9. Patients should be visually observed at all times. This can be achieved in a variety of ways.

If a central station is chosen, it should be geographically located to allow for complete visual control of all patient beds in the critical care unit. It should be designed to maximize efficiency in traffic patterns. Patients should be oriented so that they can see the nurse but cannot see the other patients. There should be an ability to communicate with the clerical staff without having to enter the central station. If a central station is not chosen, the unit should be designed to provide visual contact between patient beds so there can be constant visual contact between the nurse and patient.

A7.3.A12. To minimize distraction of those preparing medications, the area should be enclosed. A glass wall or walls may be advisable to permit visual observation of patients and unit activities. A self-contained medicine dispensing unit may be located at the nurses station, in the clean workroom, in an alcove, or in another area directly under visual control of nursing or pharmacy staff.

A7.3.A15. The recording, storage of bedside records (flowsheets, etc.), and review of clinical information is a vital function of a critical care unit. Space near the bedside for these functions should be provided. Suitable space ergonomically designed is especially germane when computers are used for the clinical record.

A7.3.A15.g. Equipment storage room or alcove. Appropriate room(s) or alcove(s) should be provided for storage of large items of equipment necessary for patient care and as required by the functional program. Its location should not interfere with the flow of traffic. Work areas and storage of critical care supplies should be in locations that are readily accessible to nursing and physician staff. Shelving, file cabinets, and drawers should be located so they are accessible to all requiring use. Separate areas need to be designed for the unit secretary and staff charting. Planning should consider the potential volume of staff (both medical and nursing) that could be present at any one time and translate that to adequate charting surfaces. The secretarial area should be accessible to all. However, the charting areas may be somewhat isolated to facilitate concentration. Storage for chart forms and supplies should be readily accessible. Space for computer terminals and printer and conduit for computer hook-up should be provided when automated information systems are in use or planned for the future. Patient records should be readily accessible to clerical, nursing, and physician staff. Alcoves should be provided for the storage and rapid retrieval of crash carts and portable monitor/defibrillator units. Grounded electrical outlets should be provided in sufficient numbers to permit recharging stored battery-operated equipment.

A7.3.D2. There should be sleeping accommodations at each child's bedside.

A7.3.D7. Space allowances for pediatric beds and cribs are greater than those required for adult beds, because of the variations in sizes and the potential for change. Adequate storage is needed to accommodate the range of supplies and equipment needed to care for children of all ages.

A7.3.E6. General lighting in the nursery should not exceed 100 footcandles measured at mattress level. The lighting fixture layout should be designed to avoid a fixture directly above or over the neonate. Whenever possible, general lighting as well as supplemental examination lights should be designed to be controlled from each incubator position. A master switch is also desirable to simultaneously control all lights in special situations.

Ambient lighting levels in newborn intensive care units (NICUs) should be adjustable through a range of at least 10 to 60 lux (approximately 1 to 60 footcandles), as measured at each bedside. Both natural and artificial light sources should have controls that allow immediate darkening of any bed position sufficient for transillumination when necessary.

Artificial light sources should have a visible spectral distribution similar to that of daylight, but should avoid unnecessary ultraviolet or infrared radiation by the use of appropriate lamps, lenses, or filters.

Separate procedure lighting should be available to each patient care station that provides no more than 1500 to 2000 lux (150 to 200 foot candles) of illumination of the patient bed. This lighting should minimize shadow and glare; it should be adjustable and highly framed so babies at adjacent bed positions will not experience an increase in illumination.

At least one source of natural light should be visible from patient care areas. External windows in patient care rooms should be glazed with appropriate materials to minimize heat gain or loss, and should be situated at least 2 feet away from any part of a patient bed to minimize radiant heat loss from the baby. All external windows should be equipped with shading devices.

A7.3.E12. At least one transition room should be provided within or immediately adjacent to the NICU that allows parents and infants extended private time together. This room should have direct, private access to sink and toilet facilities, a bed for parents, communication linkage with NICU staff, and appropriate electric and medical gas outlets. The room(s) can be used for other family educational, counseling, parent sleeping, or demonstration purposes when not needed as a transition room.

A7.3.E17. Whenever possible, supplies should flow through special supply entrances from external corridors so that penetration of the semisterile zone by non-nursery personnel is unnecessary. Soiled materials should be sealed and stored in a soiled holding area until removed. This holding area should be located where there will be no need to pass back through the semisterile zone to remove the soiled materials.

A7.4
There should be a breastfeeding/pumping room readily available for mothers of NICU babies to pump breastmilk.

A7.4.D.
When the functional program includes a mother-baby couplet approach to nursing care, the workroom functions described above may be incorporated in the nurse station that serves the postpartum patient rooms.

A7.5.
Recognizing their unique physical and developmental needs, pediatric and adolescent patients, to the extent their condition permits, should be grouped together in distinct units or distinct areas of general units separate from adults.

A7.7.B2. Separate and additional recovery space may be necessary to accommodate outpatients. If children receive care, recovery space should be provided for pediatric patients and the layout of the surgical suite should facilitate the presence of parents in the PACU.

A7.8.
Obstetrical program models vary widely in their delivery methodologies. The models are essentially three types. The following narrative describes the organizational framework of each model:

A7.8.A1. Traditional Model
Under the traditional model, labor, delivery, recovery, and postpartum occur in separate areas. The birthing woman is treated as the moving part. She is moved through these functional areas depending on the status of the birth process.

The functional areas are separate rooms consisting of the labor room, delivery room, recovery room, postpartum bedroom, and infant nurseries (levels determined by acuity).

A7.8.A2. Labor-Delivery-Recovery Model
All labor-delivery-recovery rooms (LDRs) are designed to accommodate the birthing process from labor through delivery and recovery of mother and baby. They are equipped to handle most complications, with the exception of caesarean sections.

The birthing woman moves only as a postpartum patient to her bedroom or to a caesarean section delivery room (surgical operative room) if delivery complications occur.

After the mother and baby are recovered in the LDR, they are transferred to a mother-baby care unit for postpartum stay.

A7.8.A3. Labor-Delivery-Recovery-Postpartum Model
Single room maternity care in labor-delivery-recovery-postpartum rooms (LDRPs) adds a "P" to the LDR model. Room design and capability to handle most emergencies remain the same as the LDRs. However, the LDRP model eliminates a move to postpartum after delivery. LDRP uses one private room for labor, delivery, recovery, and postpartum stay.

Equipment is moved into the room as needed, rather than moving the patient to the equipped room. Certain deliveries are handled in a caesarean section delivery room (surgical operative room) should delivery complications occur.

A7.9.A.
Classification of emergency departments/services (from the *Accreditation Manual for Hospitals,* The Joint Commission on Accreditation of Healthcare Organizations:

Level I: provides comprehensive emergency care 24 hours a day, with a physician experienced in emergency care on duty at all times. Must include in-hospital physician coverage of medical, surgical, orthopedic, obstetric/gynecologic, pediatric, and anesthesia services. Other specialty coverage must be available within approximately 30 minutes. Physical and related emotional problems must be provided in-house.

Level II: provides emergency care 24 hours a day, with a physician experienced in emergency care on duty at all times, and specialty consultation available within approximately 30 minutes. Physical and related emotional problems must be provided in-house, with transfer provisions to another facility when needed.

Level III: provides emergency care 24 hours a day, with at least one physician available within approximately 30 minutes. Specialty consultation available per medical staff request or by transfer to a designated hospital where definitive care can be provided.

Level IV: provides reasonable care in assessing if an emergency exists and in performing lifesaving first aid, with appropriate referral to the nearest hospital capable of providing needed services. Physician coverage is defined by the local medical staff.

More detailed descriptions of emergency service categories may be available from the Committee on Trauma of the American College of Surgeons and the American College of Emergency Physicians.

A7.9.C7. The need for airborne infection isolation rooms or protective environment rooms in a facility should be determined by an infection control risk assessment.

A7.9.D8. Access needs to be convenient to ambulance entrance.

A7.9.D16.a. Disposal space for regulated medical waste, e.g., gauzes/linens soaked with body fluids, should be separate from routine disposal space.

A7.9.D21. A security station and/or system should be located to maximize visibility of the treatment areas, waiting areas, and key entrance sites. This system should include visual monitoring devices installed both internally in the emergency department as well as externally at entrance sites and parking lots. Spatial requirements for a security station should include accommodation for hospital security staff, local police officers, and monitoring equipment. Design consideration should include installation of silent alarms, panic buttons, and intercom systems, and physical barriers such as doors to patient entry areas.

The security monitoring system should be included on the hospital's emergency power backup system.

A7.9.D23. A family room to provide privacy for families of critically ill or deceased patients should be located away from the main traffic and treatment areas. An enclosed room with space for comfortable seating of six to ten persons should be provided; telephone access is essential. A salon- or parlor-type ambience and incandescent lighting is preferred.

A7.9.E. Other Space Considerations

When the functional program defines the need, there should be additional space considerations as noted:

A7.9.E1. A decontamination room for both chemical and radiation exposure. This room should have a separate entrance to the emergency department, and an independent, closed drainage system. A negative airflow and ventilation system separate and distinct from the hospital system should be provided. Spatial requirements should allow for at least one stretcher, several hospital staff, two shower heads and an adjacent locked storage area for medical supplies and equipment. Solid lead-lined walls and doors should meet regulatory requirements.

A7.9.E2. A separate pediatric emergency area. This area should include space for registration, discharge, triage, waiting, and a playroom. An area for the nurse station and physician station, storage for supplies and medication, and one to two isolation rooms should also be included. Each examination/treatment room should be 100 square feet (9.29 square meters) of clear floor space, with a separate procedure/trauma room of 120 square feet (11.15 square meters) of clear floor space; each of these rooms should have handwashing facilities; vacuum, oxygen, and air outlets; examination lights; and wall/column-mounted ophthalmoscopes/otoscopes. At least one room for pelvic examinations should be included. X-ray illuminators should be available.

A7.9.E3. Observation/holding units for patients requiring observation up to 23 hours or admission to an inpatient unit. This area should be located separately but near the main emergency department. The size will depend upon the function (observation and/or holding), patient acuity mix, and projected utilization. As defined by the functional plan, this area should consist of a centralized nurse station and 100 square feet (9.29 square meters) of clear floor space for each cubicle, with vacuum, oxygen, and air outlets, monitoring space, and nurse call buttons. A patient bathroom should be provided. Storage space for medical and dietary supplies should be included. X-ray illuminators should be available.

A7.9.E4. A separate fast track area should be considered when annual emergency department visits exceed 20–30,000 visits. This area should include space for registration, discharge, triage, and waiting, as well as a physician/nurse work station. Storage areas for supplies and medication should be included. A separate treatment/procedure room of 120 square feet (11.15 square meters) of clear floor space should be provided. Examination/treatment areas should be 100 square feet (9.29 square meters) of clear floor space, with handwashing facilities; vacuum, oxygen, and air outlets; and examination lights. At least one treatment/examination room should be designated for pelvic examinations.

A7.9.E.5. A patient hygiene room with shower and toilet facilities.

A7.10.C3. Some equipment may require additional air conditioning for the computer room.

A7.10.D1. Radiography rooms should be a minimum of 180 square feet (16.72 square meters). (Dedicated chest X-ray may be smaller.)

A7.10.D2. Tomography and radiography/fluoroscopy (R&F) rooms should be a minimum of 250 square feet (23.28 square meters).

A7.10.D3. Mammography rooms should be a minimum of 100 square feet (9.29 square meters).

A7.10.E4. When provided, space should be a minimum of 50 square feet (4.65 square meters) to accommodate two large dewars of cryogen.

A7.11.F1. Space should be provided as necessary to accommodate the functional program. PET scanning is generally used in experimental settings and requires space for a scanner and for a cyclotron. The scanner room should be a minimum of 300 square feet (27.87 square meters).

A7.11.F2. Where a cyclotron room is required, it should be a minimum of 225 square feet (20.90 square meters) with a 16 square foot (4.88 square meter) space safe for storage of parts that may need to cool down for a year or more.

A7.11.F3. Both a hot (radioactive) lab and a cold (non-radioactive) lab may be required, each a minimum of 250 square feet (23.23 square meters).

A7.11.F4. A blood lab of a minimum of 80 square feet (7.43 square meters) should be provided.

A7.11.F5. A patient holding area to accommodate two stretchers should be provided.

A7.11.F6. A gas storage area large enough to accommodate bottles of gas should be provided. Each gas will be piped individually and may go to the cyclotron or to the lab. Ventilation adequate for the occupancy is required. Compressed air may be required to pressurize a water circulation system.

A7.11.F7. Significant radiation protection may be required since the cyclotron may generate high radiation.

A7.11.F8. Special ventilation systems together with monitors, sensors, and alarm systems may be required to vent gases and chemicals.

A7.11.F9. The heating, ventilating, and air conditioning system will require particular attention; highest pressures should be in coldest (radiation) areas and exhaust should be in hottest (radiation) areas. Redundancy may be important.

A7.11.F10. The cyclotron is water cooled with de-ionized water. A heat exchanger and connection to a compressor or to chilled water may be required. A redundant plumbing system connected to a holding tank may be required to prevent accidental leakage of contaminated water into the regular plumbing system.

A7.11.H4. Minimum size should be 260 square feet (24.15 square meters) for the simulator room. Minimum size, including the maze, should be 680 square feet (63.17 square meters) for accelerator rooms and 450 square feet (41.81 square meters) for cobalt rooms.

A7.12.D.
For example, separate facilities should be provided for such incompatible materials as acids and bases, and vented storage should be provided for volatile solvents.

A7.13.D4. The facilities should be similar to a residential environment.

A7.16.B.
Autopsy rooms should be equipped with downdraft local exhaust ventilation.

A7.21.A2. Clean Assembly/Workroom
Access to sterilization rooms should be restricted. This room should contain Hi-Vacuum or gravity steam sterilizers and sterilization equipment to accommodate heat-sensitive equipment (ETO sterilizer) and ETO aerators. This room is used exclusively for the inspection, assembly, and packaging of medical/surgical supplies and equipment for sterilization. Area should contain work tables, counters, a handwashing fixture, ultrasonic storage facilities for backup supplies and instrumentation, and a drying cabinet or equipment. The area should be spacious enough to hold sterilizer cars for loading of prepared supplies for sterilization.

A7.30.B2. In new construction, hospital-type elevator cars should have inside dimensions for accommodating a patient bed with attendants and equipment. Bed sizes vary depending on the type of patient served and the accessories attached to the bed. Therefore, the inside clear cab dimensions and door width should accommodate the most size-demanding type of patient bed, equipment, and staff determined by the functional program.

A7.30.C2.d. When incinerators are used, consideration should be given to the recovery of waste heat from on-site incinerators used to dispose of large amounts of waste materials.

A7.30.C2.e. Incinerators should be designed in a manner fully consistent with protection of public and environmental health, both on-site and off-site, and in compliance with federal, state, and local statutes and regulations. Toward this end, permit applications for incinerators and modifications thereof should be supported by environmental assessments and/or environmental impact statements (EISs) and/or health risk assessments (HRAs) as may be required by regulatory agencies. Except as noted below, such assessments should utilize standard U.S. EPA methods, specifically those set forth in U.S. EPA guidelines, and should be fully consistent with U.S. EPA guidelines for health risk assessment (U.S. EPA). Under some circumstances, however, regulatory agencies having jurisdiction over a particular project may require use of alternative methods.

A7.31.D6. See ACGIH Industrial Ventilation: A Manual of Recommended Practice for additional information.

A7.31.D9. One way to achieve basic humidification is to use a steam-jacketed manifold type humidifier, with a condensate separator that delivers high-quality steam. Additional booster humidification (if required) should be provided by steam jacketed humidifiers for each individually controlled area. Steam to be used for humidification may be generated in a separate steam generator. The steam generator feedwater may be supplied either from soft or reverse osmosis water. Provisions should be made for periodic cleaning.

A7.31.D24. When not performed in an airborne infection isolation room, sputum induction should be performed in an enclosed booth, with a mechanical ventilation system capable of providing at least 20 air changes per hour. The exhaust rate should be at least 50 cfm, and the space should be under negative pressure (at least 0.001" water column). The booth should contain a grille to provide make-up air that should enter with a velocity of at least 100 fpm. All air should be exhausted directly to the outside. HEPA filtration of the exhaust may be required if the exhaust point is near an outside air intake or pedestrian area.

7.31.E4.e. Floor drains in cystoscopy operating rooms have been shown to disseminate a heavily contaminated spray during flushing. Unless flushed regularly with large amounts of fluid, the trap tends to dry out and permit passage of gases, vapors, odors, insects, and vermin directly into the operating room. For new construction, if a floor drain is insisted upon by the users, the drain plate should be located away from the operative site and should be over a frequently flushed nonsplash, horizontal-flow type of bowl, preferably with a closed system of drainage. Alternative methods include (a) an aspirator/

trap installed in a wall connected to the collecting trough of the operating table by a closed, disposable tube system, or (b) a closed system using portable collecting vessels. (See NFPA 99.)

Table 2, Footnote 6. Recirculating devices with HEPA filters may have potential uses in existing facilities as interim, supplemental environmental controls to meet requirements for the control of airborne infectious agents. Limitations in design must be recognized. The design of either portable or fixed systems should prevent stagnation and short circuiting of airflow. The supply and exhaust locations should direct clean air to areas where health care workers are likely to work, across the infectious source, and then to the exhaust, so the health care worker is not in a position between the infectious source and the exhaust location. The design of such systems should also allow for easy access for scheduled preventive maintenance and cleaning.

A8.2.A. Clusters and Staffing Considerations

Clustering refers to several concepts in which the design of traditional nursing home floor plans (straight halls, double- or single-loaded corridors) is reorganized to provide benefits to the residents as well as to make the people who care for them more effective.

Clustering is done to achieve better image, faster service, shorter walking/wheeling distances, and less visible handling of linen. It can also afford more localized social areas and optional decentralized staff work areas. A functioning cluster as described here is more than an architectural form in which rooms are grouped around social areas without reference to caregiving. In a functioning cluster, the following will be accomplished:

Utility placement is better distributed for morning care: Clean and soiled linen rooms are located closer to the resident rooms, minimizing staff steps and maximizing the appearance of corridors (carts are not scattered through halls).

Unit scale and appearance reinforce the perception of smaller groups of rooms as grouped or related: Clusters should offer identifiable social groups for both staff and older people, thereby reducing the sense of largeness often associated with centralized facilities.

Geographically effective staffing: The staffing pattern and design reinforce each other so that nursing assistants can offer primary nursing care and relate to a given set of rooms. Their room assignments are grouped together and generally do not require unequal travel distances to basic utilities. Staff "buddying" is possible. Buddying involves sharing responsibilities such as lifting a non-weight bearing person, or covering for someone while the buddy provides off-unit transport, or is on a break.

Staffing that works as well at night as during the day: An effective cluster design incorporates multiple staffing ratios. A unit might have 42 beds, but with clustering could staff effectively in various ratios of licensed nurses to nurses assistants: 1:7 days (6 clusters); 1:14 or 1:21 nights (3 or 2 neighborhoods).

Clustering can also have some other benefits:

Cluster design can provide more efficient "gross/net area" when a variety of single and/or double rooms are "nested."

Cluster design can be useful when a project is to have a high proportion of private occupancy rooms, because it reduces distances to staff work areas or nursing stations.

Clusters provide a method of distributing nursing staff through a building, nearer to bedrooms at night, so they can be responsive to vocal calls for assistance and toileting. (Central placement of staff requires greater skill in using traditional call systems than many residents possess.)

Cluster units of a given size may "stack" or be placed over each other, but might have different staffing for varying care levels.

If digital call systems are used (such as those allowing reprogramming of what room reports to which zone or nursing assistant's work area), then one unit might easily be changed over time, such as when client needs justify higher ratios of nursing assistants to older people. For example, a 48-bed unit might start at 1:8 staffing but also respond to 1:6 staffing needs. In some units, staffing might also be slightly uneven, such as when 60-bed units are comprised of clusters of 1:7 and 1:8 during days.

Architectural Form and Clustering: Clusters involve architectural form and may have an impact on overall building shape. The longer length of stay of nursing home residents compared with hospital clients is one factor that makes clustering rooms in more residential groups particularly appropriate. However, the visual advantages of units without long corridors has also attracted hospital planners. In both facility types, architectural clustering may help both staff and residents socially identify a space or subunit within a larger unit.

Though architectural clustering may involve grouping rooms, this should not happen at the expense of windowless social areas or the incorporation of all social options in a windowless social area directly outside of bedroom doorways.

A8.2.C1. Whether centralized or decentralized, staff work areas should be designed to minimize the institutional character, command-station appearance, and noise associated with traditional medical nursing stations and foster close, open relationships between residents and staff. Confidentiality or noisy staff conversations should be accommodated in an enclosed staff lounge and/or conference area. At least part of each staff work area should be low enough and open enough to permit easy conversations between staff and residents seated in wheelchairs.

A8.3.A.
It is important to provide outdoor views from dining, recreation, and living spaces.

A8.4.
Activities programs focus on the social, spiritual, and creative needs of residents and clients and provide quality, meaningful experiences for them. These programs may be facility-wide or for smaller groups.

If included in the functional program, the Activities department is generally responsible for coordination of activities for large groups, as well as small groups and personalized individual programs involving one resident and one therapist. These activities may be conducted in other portions of the building (e.g., dining rooms, recreation spaces, lounges, etc.), but dedicated spaces are preferred for efficient operation of quality programs. Large space requirements (e.g., libraries, chapels, auditoriums, and conference, classroom, and/or training spaces) are incumbent upon the programming decisions of the sponsors as reflected in the functional program for the facility.

A8.4.B1. If required by the functional program, include space for files, records, computers, and administrative activities; a storage space for supplies and equipment;, and a quiet space for residents to converse. This quiet space may be incorporated within space for administrative activities.

Note: Hearing loss in the elderly is well documented. Quiet space is very important to enable conversation.

A8.6.
Consideration should be given to the special ventilation and exhaust requirements of these areas.

A8.7
This text is included in the appendix to solicit future public proposals to help the committee develop minimum guidelines for this service and facility type.

Subacute Services: Struggling to Define the Continuum

Most observers consider subacute care a loophole in the prospective payment system. So, it comes as no surprise that health care providers eagerly initiate discussion about this nontraditional level of care. However, these discussions have become the source of much conflict as each provider group works to create its own concept of subacute services.

Exceptions can be found to any definition of subacute care, which is also called transitional care, post-acute care, and skilled care, depending on the type of provider. Only if a separate definition is developed for each type of provider does a clear definition of subacute services begin to emerge.

With that in mind, groups seeking to develop subacute services must agree on a working definition for their organization. Currently, subacute services are found in four types of facilities, each of which has a different model of care for a different patient mix. These include acute care hospitals, rehabilitation hospitals, nursing homes, and subacute facilities.

Acute care hospitals generally provide subacute services in a physically distinct unit with beds certified by Medicare as skilled nursing facility (SNF) beds. The unit is used for patients who continue to require medical supervision at a level higher than that provided for nursing home patients but less than that required in a medical/surgical bed.

Rehabilitation hospitals may provide subacute care to several different patient groups. Patients who are ready for discharge from an acute care hospital, but who do not meet the admissions criteria for intensive rehabilitation, may receive subacute care at a rehabilitation hospital. Others may be admitted for a short stay during which rehabilitation services are provided, but not at the intensity provided to those admitted for acute rehabilitation services. Finally, patients who have completed an intensive rehabilitation program may receive subacute services when they no longer need the same intensity of therapies but are not yet ready for discharge home.

A significant shift is noted among the services of nursing homes, which are providing more skilled nursing and rehabilitation services than those traditionally found at these facilities. Distinct units are certified by Medicare as SNFs. Diagnoses are similar to those found in a SNF in an acute care hospital. However, because of the differences in overhead, care can be provided at markedly lower costs.

Specialty subacute facilities are the newest players on the block. These are generally developed by entrepreneurs capitalizing on a unique and profitable niche in the health care industry. They may be licensed as acute care hospitals or as specialty hospitals. Patients generally represent those who require intensive care services for an extended period, including catastrophic illness and post-surgery. These patients are classified as subacute because of the long-term nature of their acute medical conditions.

A8.8.A.
The latest edition of the Life Safety Code recognizes the need to lock doors in Alzheimer's units. Consideration should be given to making locks on wardrobes, closets, or cupboards inconspicuous.

A8.8.B.
Outdoor spaces may include gardens on grade or on roof decks, or solaria, porches, balconies, etc. Lounge space may be a winterized sunroom, a designated lounge space separate from the dining room, or a dayroom, where other residents may be sitting. Secure, accessible outdoor space can provide a calming change in environment and also a convenient place for agitated residents to walk.

A8.8.C.
Major characteristics of persons with Alzheimer's and other dementias are lack of attention span and an inability to orient themselves within space. The environment should provide attention-grabbing landmarks and wayfinding cues and information to aid in navigation from point to point. Sensory cuing used in other long-term care resident areas should be incorporated for persons with dementia. Dementia program activities may include memory stimulation, music therapy, art therapy, horticultural therapy, etc. Space for dining and activities in dedicated dementia units may be provided within the unit, or directly accessible to the residents of the unit, per the minimum standards described elsewhere in Chapter 8.

A8.8.C1. Landmarks: Design elements that provide clear reference points in the environment, e.g., a room, a large three-dimensional object, large picture, or other wall-mounted artifact.

A8.8.C2. Signs: When appropriate, large characters and redundant word/picture combinations should be used on signs.

A8.8.C3. Environmental design challenge: Residents with mental impairment often find it difficult to sit for long periods of time or to sit at all without becoming restless. Although it is not a universal trait, it is so common and requires so much staff time that environmental solutions should be explored in all areas, to give cognitively impaired people interesting places and things on which to focus their attention.

A8.14.
Hot surfaces are intended to include those surfaces to which residents have normal access and exceed 110°F. This requirement does not intend to include medical or therapeutic equipment.

A8.14.A5. Where local requirements permit, wire-free, fire-rated safety glazing should be used to enhance the homelike residential appearance preferred by residents and visitors.

A8.14.A7. Consideration should be given to increasing clearances for arthritic residents.

A8.15.A8. Consideration should be given to increasing clearances for arthritic residents and for mounting handrails lower than required by ADA, to enable frail residents to lean on the handrails for support when ambulating.

A8.30.B2. Handrail projections of up to 3.5 inches (8.89 centimeters) should not be construed as diminishing the clear inside dimensions.

A8.31.D1. ASHRAE Standard 55 recommends 30 to 60 percent relative humidity for comfort. In cold or arid climates, achieving relative humidities as high as 30 percent may not be practical. Where central ventilation systems are not utilized, these humidity requirements may not be achievable. Additional data are needed to establish a consensus on the cost/benefit of maintaining humidity within the recommended range.

If duct humidifiers are located upstream of the final filters, they should be located at least 15 feet (4.56 meters) upstream of the final filters. Ductwork with duct-mounted humidifiers located downstream of the final filters should have a means of water removal. An adjustable high-limit humidistat should be located downstream of the humidifier to reduce the potential for condensation inside the duct. All duct takeoffs should be sufficiently downstream of the humidifier to ensure complete moisture absorption. Steam humidifiers should be used. Reservoir-type water spray or evaporative pan humidifiers should not be used.

Exhaust hoods handling grease-laden vapors in food preparation centers should comply with NFPA 96. All hoods over cooking ranges should be equipped with grease filters, fire extinguishing systems, and heat-actuated fan controls. Cleanout openings should be provided every 20 feet (6.10 meters) and at changes in direction in the horizontal exhaust duct systems serving these hoods. (Horizontal runs of ducts serving range hoods should be kept to a minimum.)

A8.31.D8. It is recommended that when practical, ventilation requirements be met by a central air handling system with filtration and humidification provisions. This system may be designed for ventilation only, with heating and cooling accomplished by non-central air handling equipment (e.g., fan coil units, heat pumps, etc.). These non-central units should be equipped with permanent, cleanable or replaceable filters with a minimum efficiency of 68 percent weight arrestance. For ventilation purposes, these units may be used as recirculating units only.

A8.32.A4a. The reader should refer to the *IES Lighting Handbook* and *Lighting for Health Care Facilities* for additional information.

A8.32.A4.b. Excessive differences in lighting levels should be avoided in transition areas between parking lots, building entrances, and lobbies or corridors; in transition zones between driveways and parking garages; etc. As the eye ages, pupils become smaller and less elastic, making visual adaptation to dark spaces slower. Upon entering a space with a considerably lower lighting level, elderly residents may need to stop or move to one side until their eyes adapt to excessive lighting changes. Elderly pedestrians may need several minutes to adjust to significant changes in brightness when entering a building from a sunlit walkway or terrace.

Consideration should be given to increasing both indoor and outdoor illumination levels in such transition spaces to avoid excessive differences between electric lighting levels and natural daytime and nighttime illumination levels. In addition, it is very helpful for pedestrians to have conveniently located places to wait, giving them time to adjust their eyes to different lighting environments. Seating areas off busy lobbies or corridors can minimize the potential for accidents by giving them the extra time they need.

Care should be taken to minimize extremes of brightness within spaces and in transitions between spaces. Excessive brightness contrast from windows or lighting systems can disorient residents.

Lighting that creates glare and colors that do not differentiate between horizontal and vertical planes, or between objects and their backgrounds (such as handrails or light switches from walls, hardware from doors, faucets from sinks, or control knobs from appliances), should be avoided, unless therapeutic benefits can be demonstrated. (For example, it has been demonstrated that deliberately camouflaged door hardware may help control wandering and elopements by some cognitively impaired residents in Alzheimer's care facilities.)

A.8.32.A4.c. Care should be taken to avoid injury from lighting fixtures. Light sources that may burn residents or ignite bed linen by direct contact should be covered or protected.

Determination of average illuminance on a horizontal plane from general lighting only. The use of this method in the types of areas described should result in values of average illuminance within 10 percent of the values that would be obtained by dividing the area into 2-foot (0.6-meter) squares, taking a reading in each square, and averaging.

The measuring instrument should be positioned so that when readings are taken, the surface of the light sensitive cell is in a horizontal plane and 30 inches (760 millimeters) above the floor. This can be facilitated by means of a small portable stand of wood or other material that will support the cell at the correct height and in the proper plane. Daylight may be excluded during illuminance measurements. Readings can be taken at night or with shades, blinds, or other opaque covering on the fenestration.

Table 6, Footnote 10. Recirculating devices with HEPA filters may have potential uses in existing facilities as interim, supplemental environmental controls to meet requirements for the control of airborne infectious agents. Limitations in design must be recognized. The design of either portable or fixed systems should prevent stagnation and short-circuiting of airflow. The supply and exhaust locations should direct clean air to areas where health care workers are likely to work, across the infectious source, and then to the exhaust, so that the health care worker is not in a position between the infectious source and the exhaust location. The design of such systems should also allow for easy access for scheduled preventive maintenance and cleaning.

A9.3.F.
Examination rooms and services as described in Section 9.2.B may be provided. In addition, offices and/or practitioner consultation rooms may be combined with examination rooms.

A9.7.
The birthing center was conceptualized as small (intimate), homelike service units serving a population of healthy childbearing families approaching pregnancy and birthing as a normal family event and seeking care in a safe environment outside of, but with access to, the acute-care hospital setting when needed. The freestanding birthing center may be a separate outpatient facility.

A9.8.A.
The range of services provided in these facilities is very dynamic and growing, including diagnostic cardiac catheterization, general radiography, fluoroscopy, mammography, CT scanning, magnetic resonance imaging (MRI), ultrasound, radiation therapy, and IV therapies. Facilities may specialize in only one of these areas or may provide a mix of services.

A9.9.A1. Wall outlets should be planned to minimize exposed power cords and cables. Monitors should be located to provide practitioners with an optimal view.

A9.30.C2.d When incinerators are used, consideration should be given to the recovery of waste heat from on-site incinerators used to dispose of large amounts of waste materials.

A9.30.C2.e Incinerators should be designed in a manner fully consistent with protection of public and environmental health, both on-site and off-site, and in compliance with federal, state, and local statutes and regulations. Toward this end, permit applications for incinerators and modifications thereof should be supported by environmental assessments and/or environmental impact statements (EISs) and/or health risk assessments (HRAs) as may be required by regulatory agencies. Except as noted below, such assessments should utilize standard U.S. EPA methods, specifically those set forth in U.S. EPA guidelines, and should be fully consistent with U.S. EPA guidelines for health risk assessment (U.S. EPA). Under some circumstances, however, regulatory agencies having jurisdiction over a particular project may require use of alternative methods.

A9.31.D6. See ACGIH Industrial Ventilation: A Manual of Recommended Practice for additional information.

A9.31.D9. One way to achieve basic humidification is with a steam-jacketed manifold type humidifier, with a condensate separator that delivers high-quality steam. Additional booster humidification (if required) can be provided by steam-jacketed humidifiers for each individually controlled area. Steam to be used for humidification may be generated in a separate steam generator. The steam generator feedwater may be supplied either from soft or reverse osmosis water. Provisions should be made for periodic cleaning.

A9.31.D22. When not performed in an airborne infection isolation room, sputum induction should be performed in an enclosed booth with a mechanical ventilation system capable of providing at least 20 air changes per hour. The exhaust rate should be at least 50 cfm, and the space should be under negative pressure (at least 0.001" water column). The booth should contain a grille to provide make-up air that should enter with a velocity of at least 100 fpm. All air should be exhausted directly to the outside. HEPA filtration of the exhaust may be required, if the exhaust point is near an outside air intake or pedestrian area.

A10.31.D5. One way to achieve basic humidification is with a steam jacketed manifold type humidifier, with a condensate separator that delivers high-quality steam. Additional booster humidification (if required) should be provided by steam-jacketed humidifiers for each individually controlled area. Steam to be used for humidification may be generated in a separate steam generator. The steam generator feedwater may be supplied either from soft or reverse osmosis water. Provisions should be made for periodic cleaning.

A10.31.D17. When not performed in an airborne infection isolation room, sputum induction should be performed in an enclosed booth with a mechanical ventilation system capable of providing at least 20 air changes per hour. The exhaust rate should be at least 50 cfm, and the space should be under negative pressure (at least 0.001" water column). The booth should contain a grille to provide make-up air that should enter with a velocity of at least 100 fpm. All air should be exhausted directly to the outside. HEPA filtration of the exhaust may be required, if the exhaust point is near an outside air intake or pedestrian area.

A11.9.D5. Exposure to some art materials, such as solvents and ceramic glazes, is associated with adverse health effects. Such risks should be controlled by adopting methods recommended in appropriate instructional manuals.

A11.9.D8. Display areas for patients' work such as shelves or wall surfaces should be provided.

A11.30.C2.d. When incinerators are used, consideration should be given to the recovery of waste heat from on-site incinerators used to dispose of large amounts of waste materials.

A11.30.C2.e. Incinerators should be designed in a manner fully consistent with protection of public and environmental health, both on-site and off-site, and in compliance with federal, state, and local statutes and regulations. Toward this end, permit applications for incinerators and modifications thereof should be supported by environmental assessments and/or environmental impact statements (EISs) and/or health risk assessments (HRAs) as may be required by regulatory agencies. Except as noted below, such assessments should utilize standard U.S. EPA methods, specifically those set forth in U.S. EPA guidelines, and should be fully consistent with U.S. EPA guidelines for health risk assessment (U.S. EPA). Under some circumstances, however, regulatory agencies having jurisdiction over a particular project may require use of alternative methods.

A11.31.D5. See ACGIH Industrial Ventilation: A Manual of Recommended Practice for additional information.

A11.31.D14. When not performed in an airborne infection isolation room, sputum induction should be performed in an enclosed booth, with a mechanical ventilation system capable of providing at least 20 air changes per hour. The exhaust rate should be at least 50 cfm, and the space should be under negative pressure (at least 0.001" water column). The booth should contain a grille to provide make-up air that should enter with a velocity of at least 100 fpm. All air should be exhausted directly to the outside. HEPA filtration of the exhaust may be required, if the exhaust point is near an outside air intake or pedestrian area.

A13. Hospice Care

This text is added to the appendix to solicit public comment.

To improve the quality of life for terminally ill individuals, their caregivers, families, and loved ones, hospices are becoming increasingly important alternative environments and/or alternative care systems. Hospice facilities are being developed in acute care hospitals, as part of nursing facilities, and as freestanding facilities, with little available guidance as to which functional elements and environmental features are necessary and appropriate. Available books and publications address the rationales and philosophies that motivate hospice care providers. However, no research-based guidelines for hospice design and/or construction currently exist.

Many hospice facilities built to date have been renovations of parts of existing hospital or nursing care facilities. As such, they are too full of compromise to serve as adequate guides to the future of hospice design.

Form for Proposals on AIA Guidelines for Design and Construction of Hospital and Health Care Facilities

Date

Name

Organization

Address

Telephone

Fax

All proposals must refer to specific parts of the 1996-97 edition of the Guidelines. Each separate proposal requires a separate copy of this form. Only proposals that appear on this form, and that are received during a formal proposal submittal period (to be publicly announced), can be considered.

1. Section/paragraph: _____ Page no.: _____

2. Proposal recommends (check one):
   new text   _____
   revised text   _____
   deleted text   _____

3. Proposals (include new, revised, or wording to be deleted):

4. Statement of problem and substantiation for proposal:

Use additional sheets if necessary; attach all documentation to this form.

Mail to:
   Academy of Architecture for Health
   American Institute of Architects
   1735 New York Avenue, N.W.
   Washington, D.C. 20006

I agree to give AIA all and full rights, including rights of copyright, in this proposal and I understand that I acquire no rights in any publication of AIA in which this proposal in this manner or similar or analogous form is used.

Signature

NOTARI ASSOCIATES, PA
190 W. Ostend Street
Suite 110
Baltimore, MD 21230

NOTARI ASSOCIATES, PA
190 W. Ostend Street
Suite 110
Baltimore, MD 21230